Your Tastebuds Are A**holes

D1516119

Your Tastebuds Are A**holes

How I Trained Mine and Healed Crohn's

Unique Hammond

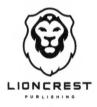

LIONCREST
PUBLISHING

YOUR TASTEBUDS ARE A**HOLES

How I Trained Mine and Healed Crohn's

ISBN   978-1-5445-1022-4 *Paperback*
       978-1-5445-1023-1 *Ebook*

Dedicated to those who believed in my journey and supported me through my darkest hours and to those who are just beginning theirs. I believe in you.

Contents

· · · · · · ·

"The only way to keep your health is to eat what you don't want, drink what you don't like, and do what you'd rather not."

—MARK TWAIN

Introduction

Your Taste Buds Are Assholes

. . . .

I know what you're thinking:

How dare I insult your taste buds by calling them assholes?

It's true, I've never met your amazing, beautiful, life-enhancing taste buds. I'm sure they are fantastical, along with all the taste memories they have ushered into your life. (Except, perhaps, for the "getting drunk on tequila and vomiting all night into your hair" memory. Yuck.)

They're your taste buds, and you know them best. But here's something you may not know:

While your taste buds are taking you on this magic carpet ride of sensory pleasure, they are distracting you from what is really going on inside your body.

Have you ever found yourself running to the market in your pajamas in search of ice cream? Or hitting the drive-through after dinner? Or ransacking the fridge at 2:00 a.m. for the treats you made for your kid's school holiday party? The culprit? It's your asshole taste buds. (Or being totally stoned. These days, it could easily be both.)

Believe it or not, your taste buds are trying to kill you. And no lawyer can prosecute them.

Why'd You Have to Go and Make Things So Complicated?

There was a time, long before you and I were ever born, when eating was simple. People woke up with the sun, went off to hunt and gather, came back to share and consume what they had, and went to sleep knowing they'd do it all over again the next day.

Today, however, we have an infinite variety of delectable options available to us—no hunting or gathering required. With all this constant abundance, how do we choose what to eat? Our taste buds are ready with an answer: whatever tastes the best!

Particularly true in the Western world, more importance is placed on flavor versus content. But while flavor delights your taste buds, most of the time it does nothing for the rest of your body. (You know, that thing that drags your mouth around.) And the more you indulge your taste buds, the more bossy they get, until they turn into entitled little brats that reject anything that doesn't come covered in sugar or melted cheese. (I'm looking at you, happy hour.)

With food allergies and autoimmune disorders on the rise, our bodies need us more than ever to get our spoiled asshole taste buds in line. We need to treat our taste buds like a well-loved child. We need to give them what they need, not what they want. We need to train the asshole out of them. Our lives literally depend on it.

If I could live in a dream, I would eat marshmallows, drink coffee with cream, eat a doughnut with a dash of brandy (in the coffee of course) all day long...and at the end of that amazing day, I would swim in a vat of my favorite tequila. Ahhhh.

But life is not a dream, especially not when you're living it as a slave to your asshole taste buds. Life is as real as stomach issues, uncontrollable farting, and bad breath. My apologies if you didn't know that. But if you're reading this book, my guess is that you already do.

My Journey, My Story

After spending three years battling Crohn's disease, I'm definitely not short on opinions when it comes to health and longevity. (Just ask my friends and family.) However, I do believe that everyone's health is their own journey, and that journey is made up of the steps they choose to take.

I've written this book to give you a picture of my journey and the choices I made—both the choices that led to my disease, and the choices that brought about my surprising recovery—in the hope of helping you begin the health journey that is right for you.

By learning to retrain my bossy, entitled taste buds, I was able to regain my health. I not only healed my autoimmune disease, but I've continued to thrive against all the dire prognoses doctors gave me...with no drugs, surgery, or crazy rules around food other than eat well.

One of the worst things autoimmune diseases like Crohn's can do to you is turn food into a boogeyman. This isn't a book about how to go from being a taste bud asshole to a food asshole. Believe me when I say that I do indeed enjoy a hamburger here and a tequila there. But, more importantly, I enjoy eating for longevity of my badass health.

Food is simple; we're the ones who make it complicated.

In the following pages, you're going to rediscover how easily food can help you maintain optimal health or, if you are in bad shape like I was, how to regain your health and feel more alive than ever.

Being Healthy Is the Opposite of Being Deprived

A lot of people think making changes to live a healthier life means deprivation or becoming a California health nut (like me). They don't want to have to change their routine. They don't want to have to give up their favorite foods. Or be different or explain why they don't eat shit and get wasted on the weekend.

I was never an overweight person. I made sure to control my portions, and, when I felt like I'd been "bad," I would eat a salad to compensate. When you came right down to it, my body was made of what I ate on a whim, what I was "craving," instead of what it needed. I didn't know this at the time; I was oblivious.

The sad fact is that you usually can't trust what tastes good. Why? Because amazing chefs and food scientists have figured out how to engineer those umami flavors that we crave, along with junk food companies whose only aim is for you to buy more, more, more. Your favorite fast food or packaged snack has been scientifically created so that you can't stop eating it.

Scary, right?

When you think about it that way, it's easy to see that health is not about deprivation. Quite the contrary. It's about loving yourself so much that living a full, joyous, satisfying life is the standard. Living for health and well-being requires that you contemplate health on a cellular level that comes from—surprise!—feeding your body healthy, unprocessed proteins and fats instead of simple, heavily processed carbs and sugars. It means looking past your "fast metabolism" or slender build and making sure you're building a healthy body on a cellular level that you can live in, comfortably and happily, until you're ready to depart planet Earth.

We Really Are What We Eat

I lived a huge chunk of my adult life in constant pain from Crohn's disease. It came out of nowhere like a sucker punch to the face. In the beginning, I didn't know what was wrong with me. I just knew something was wrong. I also knew deep down inside that there was something out there that could heal me—I just had to find it. My journey was a needle-in-a-haystack kind of journey.

Needless to say, after nearly every doctor visit I had, I left feeling broken. Unfixable, really. I felt like the only thing available to me were a bunch of "Band-Aids," things to make me "comfortable" with my disease that I'd be living with for the rest of my life. (As if.) There was nobody along the way that made me feel like my life could get back to being great, like it used to be. To me, that was incredibly disheartening.

Doctors are wonderful when it comes to saving your life in an emergency, or giving you tests that reveal exactly what has gone haywire. Family is great for emotional support and offering sympathy (if you're lucky). In the end, however, only *you* can be an advocate for your own health. I know—sucks, right? I think we all secretly hope that someone else will save us when we mess up; it's a tough pill to swallow realizing that every unhealthy choice you stuff into your mouth or inject into your body plays a part in your disease story.

So, I beg you, before you make the irreversible decision to cut and remove parts of yourself, ask yourself some real questions:

- What changes can I make today that will support my body being healthy?
- How can I live in a way that is more respectful of this amazing body that I've been given?

- How can I avoid having a doctor show me how to fix a problem that I have co-created?

Above all, you must ask yourself whether it's worth letting your life be run by your asshole taste buds.

This book is going to show you that natural healing is possible. Bear in mind, though, that natural healing takes time and patience. I heard a doctor once say that for every year you're sick, it takes a month to heal. My experience was different: for every month I was sick, it took two months to heal.

It also takes commitment—healing through food doesn't work when you only make good choices half the time. You'll need to drop your excuses and put on your big girl boots for this ride.

By sharing my story, I want to not only counsel you on the healing path, but help you be patient with it. It's a call to awareness, of your body, your vehicle through life, and to help you create some goals for that.

Along with the healing diet I'm going to teach, this book is meant to provide a real human perspective into healing through a nonclinical approach. I want to provide a window into my trial-and-error process, so you see where my results really came from. A lot of things out there are written by people who haven't necessarily dealt with Crohn's personally. I know I discovered that with nutritionists—they were trying to help me, they should have had all the information, but without having firsthand experience of it, they couldn't really provide me what I needed to overcome that mountain. If they did, everybody would be doing nutrition over prescription! A lot of the books I read were very clinical, hard to read, and frankly, not inspiring.

When you're choosing to heal naturally, a lot of people will remind you that this approach is against the odds. I've written this book to help you say, "Screw 'em," and keep on doing right by your body.

I'm here to be your personal cheerleader and champion. I'll be reminding you that no matter how shitty you feel and how messed up your life looks right now, you're great. And you have even more greatness within you. Your body is on your side and wants to help you heal. You might feel weak today, but you have everything you need to climb out of the shit. All it takes is some education, dedication, hope, and a sense of humor. Let's do this together.

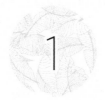

1

You're Great

. . . .

"Mom, can I help you with that?" My eldest daughter stood in the doorway of the kitchen, saying the words every mother loves to hear—every mother except me on that morning.

I'd spent another sleepless night moaning and rocking back and forth through bouts of excruciating pain. My eyes were baggy; my head felt filled with sand. The only positive was, when the sun would rise, sometimes the pain subsided to a dull ache. However, I knew it would be back. It always came back. Stupid pain.

All I wanted was to make breakfast for my kids, but even the smallest motions—pulling out the pan, breaking eggs, standing at the stove while stirring—happened in slow motion. The pain increased, radiating up my back and into my neck. With every moment I stood at the stove, fiery pressure mounted in my stomach, my joints, and my gut. My entire body tensed, bracing against the pain. I couldn't take it; I had to sit down. After a few shallow breaths, I got back up, stirred a little longer, only to take a seat again. The pain was too much.

This is how my sweet daughter found me. She knew without asking what was happening, and she knew there was nothing she could do. So, she said the one thing she could think of:

"Mom? Can I help?"

I nodded yes, but inside I thought, *No—not this. I want my girls to help me carry grocery bags, mop the floor, or work beside me in the garden. This is where I get to be a mom. I don't want help with this. I don't want to need anyone's help with this.*

I was devastated beyond words. Pain was one thing, but being unable to scramble eggs for my girls' breakfast was humiliating.

This was where Crohn's disease had brought me, to my knees.

A Bad Place, and How I Got There

Looking back, the disease was on its way long before it took over my life. Throughout my twenties, I struggled with transient stomach issues, but I always blamed it on something I ate that just "didn't agree with me." But over time, those transient stomach issues turned into a way of life. By the time I entered my thirties, stomach pain and nausea were taking up more and more of my days, making me unable to keep down food and water, and keeping me up at night.

I was in a bad place; worse than that, I was dragging everyone I loved down with me. A sustained illness affects everything about your life, and as a parent, it's a very difficult thing to share with a family. I did my best to keep it together around my husband and children, but they knew. They saw me rocking back and forth, a motion that weirdly eased the pain. They sometimes found me curled up sobbing on the bathroom floor, or passed out and bent double on the couch. The pain and suffering were often beyond my control to hide.

My girls were young then, ages seven and ten. Despite being involved in their own lives—sports, school, friends— it was concerning for them to see their mom constantly in pain. They'd come to visit me in my bedroom, lie beside me and talk about their day. I wished that I could explain what I was going through to them, but it wasn't something they could understand. Even I didn't understand what was wrong with me.

I went to many doctors, who looked at many different possibilities—bacterial infections, gallstones, gallbladder disease, parasites—to figure out what was wrong with me. I tried every kind of remedy, from traditional approaches like antibiotics, to holistic approaches such as acupuncture, to some esoteric stuff such as kinesiology (a.k.a., muscle testing). Throughout it all, I tried to fend off the desperation that came from this faceless, daunting pain.

In 2010, I agreed to do a colonoscopy. I took the sedative, went under, and came up to a firm diagnosis: severe Crohn's disease. I was surprised at how relieved I felt afterward—naming the disease had been my biggest fear. But the relief quickly faded as the doctors began to go through the available options for dealing with it. If you've ever dealt with Crohn's (and if you're reading this book, you're probably dealing with it right now), you already know what I learned at that time: none of your options are good.

My Life Before and After

Before Crohn's, I was happy, hardworking, passionate

about my life and my family. I loved trail running, kite-boarding, and surfing. I traveled all over the country for my job. I was deeply invested in my daughters' lives, helping them grow and celebrating their milestones.

Over the course of five years, Crohn's disease sapped all the joy and passion from my life. I could not feel the same emotions I used to. All I could feel was pain, twenty-four hours a day.

The best days were the ones the pain would subside to mere discomfort. It was as if the sun had come out in my life—I could enjoy listening to my daughters' stories, I could get out of bed, hobble about, and cook for my family. Oh, the joy of being somewhat normal, even if just for an hour or so...who knew being normal was such a gift?

Before long, though, the clouds would close back over me. The severe pain would return, and I'd retreat to my bed where, if I was lucky, I'd get about twenty minutes of broken sleep before the excruciating pain would punch me in the gut.

Determined to Heal

I recently looked back at photos of my family from a visit we made to my hometown of Big Sur. I often dodged the camera during my illness—the person I saw in the photographs wasn't me—but somehow, I got caught in a few photos during that trip. I'm still shocked by how I look in those photos—a grown woman, her glassy eyes filled with pain, wearing jeans the size of her pre-teen daughters'. On me, they hung loose.

I'd shrunk down to ninety pounds at my sickest, yet hardly anyone who saw me recognized something was wrong. That's life in Los Angeles for you—everywhere I went, people told me I looked great. I remember thinking, "How is this possible? How are people not seeing me? How are they thinking being this skinny is healthy?"

Still, I kept pushing myself to keep my life going. I continued to work and even traveled often, sometimes despite my husband's protests. During the weeks that I was unable to get out of bed, I'd drag my laptop onto my swollen belly and work from my bedroom, taking and making calls. I was determined to not let my life be dictated by my illness.

Doctors

After my official diagnosis, I was convinced all I had to do was find the right way to support my body so it could be healthy. For a period of about six months, I saw a series of doctors. Some prescribed painkillers for me, from Percocet to Vicodin, and, of course, the catchall Nexium for my acid reflux. Most wanted me on immune suppressants for eternity.

This was not the advice I wanted to hear. First, I'm overly sensitive to medications. Alcohol and Advil affect me more than the average person. I was afraid of the damage these painkillers might inflict on my weak body. It didn't make sense to numb the pain instead of dealing with the root cause.

Second, it made no sense to me that the solution to my pain was to cut out part of my body or cover up the problem with prescription medications. If a bee stung your finger, you wouldn't cut off your hand. I didn't want to lose a piece of my body; I wanted my body to be strong as a whole. The idea of playing "whack-a-mole" with my intestines—every time the inflammation showed up, either cutting it out or taking a new drug when the old one stopped working? NOT A CHANCE.

When I saw doctors, I was clear with them: my goal was to heal my illness, not cover it up. That meant not living with part of my intestines gone, not depending on medication, and certainly not "healing" my disease by creating another one. When they tried to sell me on tests or treatments, saying, "The odds are so small—one person in a thousand has complications," I'd nod and politely decline. I did not want to be that one person. I loved life too much to risk it on a solution that might do more harm than good in the long run.

Drugs

At one point, when I became alarmingly emaciated, I got desperate enough to go on a five-week course of Prednisone, an anti-inflammatory drug.

Taking Prednisone felt like black magic. Not only did it make my pain disappear, but it gave me a mental and emotional reprieve from the daily agony. However, it also brought a crazy, manic energy I had never felt before. While I was on it, I ate ravenously and kept food down. I'd walk the hills around my house feeling invincible, like the Terminator. However, I knew in the back of my mind there was a price to pay for this "miracle" cure. I'd done the research on Prednisone and knew it wasn't beneficial for your long-term health. It weakens the immune system and prevents our bodies from getting all the nutrients they should from the food we consume. No bueno. I knew I couldn't stay on it, even though there were moments I wished I could. It temporarily brought me back to life.

At the end of five weeks, I went off Prednisone. Sure

enough, the pain quickly returned as the inflammation awakened from its premature sleep. Without healing the core issue, the fire in my intestines raged on beneath the Band-Aid.

Diets

Deep down inside, I was convinced that food had to play a major role in how I would get better. While my family slept, I spent my nights rocking back and forth, quietly moaning in pain while Googling every possible diet that promised to heal autoimmune disorders like mine. First, I went through the elimination diet, where you omit foods that commonly cause allergic or digestive reactions—wheat, dairy, soy, sugar, eggs, nuts, etc. When that didn't change anything, I tried the low-residue diet designed to reduce the frequency and volume of stools, while prolonging intestinal transit time. This included restricting foods that increased bowel activity, such as whole grains, fruits, and veggies.

> "Residue" refers to undigested foods, mostly fiber, hanging around in the colon.

Next, there was the specific carbohydrate diet, which has helped millions of people with various forms of bowel disease. The gluten-free diet, the paleo diet, the macrobiotic diet—I tried them all, and to my great sadness, none of them worked for me. WTF.

The Last Diet I'd Ever Try

One day, a friend called and said she wanted to drop off a book she thought might have information that could help me. This was something people did from time to time—bring me resources they thought might help. Most often they would email me healing recipes, articles about Crohn's breakthroughs and even poop transplants. Yummy.

I appreciated their eagerness to help, and felt blessed to be so loved. Sometimes I would try some of the remedies they suggested. But with Crohn's, anything can send you into an outright crazy flare. In other words, trying random diets or supplements wasn't the best idea.

Even though people cared about me, nobody could really understand what I was going through. Crohn's disease is a very personal illness. Not only is it all about the stuff you're taught to not talk about (i.e., poop issues), but it also shows up differently for each person. The very nature of Crohn's is that your body is too inflamed to heal the way other people do, through taking in nutrition and eliminating waste. It's a disease that makes you feel completely alone.

Once my friend left, I hobbled outside and grabbed the book she'd left for me. But I barely looked at it. In fact, I threw it across the room and forgot about it. Later, though, curiosity got the better of me. I picked it up and studied the front cover of this latest resource.

This one had a different angle from anything I'd seen before. It was by a woman named Karen Hurd, a pastor's wife in Wisconsin, who had developed this diet to help her family after they experienced autoimmune issues similar to mine. After successfully healing her family with this diet, she'd gone on to help a great number of people who called her with all kinds of autoimmune illnesses—rheumatoid arthritis, ulcerative colitis, and yes, even Crohn's disease.

The healing ingredient in this diet? It was the last thing I'd ever have expected. It was, in my opinion at that time, one of the most difficult foods to digest, and I would be bat shit crazy to try it. It sounded not only improbable, but unappetizing. (In Chapter 4 I go into the diet in detail, in case you want to skip ahead to find out the mystery ingredient.)

The book was titled *They Said It Wasn't Possible*. When I read that, I thought, *No shit, it's not possible*. The thought was followed by another: *Do I have it in me to try one more diet?* At this point I was three-plus years into my hellish health journey, and felt physically, emotionally, and mentally beat-up.

Despite my cynicism at that point, the success stories in this book were impossible to ignore, and I couldn't stifle the hope I felt building in my soul. The pages of Karen's book told of patient after patient who, after following her protocol, got better. And the plain fact was that I had no other options left at this point, except to become a "lab rat" trying different medications in hopes of finding one that worked. I didn't want to get my hopes up again. I didn't want to try yet another "miracle" diet that would fail me. But I was desperate to heal. *So,* I thought, *here goes nothing.*

I finished the book on a Friday night. On Saturday, I started the diet. The following Tuesday, I called Karen in Wisconsin for a consultation, and began my journey of healing.

And you know what? That crazy book with its crazy diet changed my life.

Hope for Healing

To my great surprise, a few weeks into Karen's diet—which I took to calling the Desperation Diet—my pain started to subside. As the weeks passed, I began experiencing one, then two, then several hours at a time without pain.

Eventually, those hours turned into days. Eventually, those days crowded together and made weeks. Whole weeks without pain or nausea. It was like a dream. The world looks different without constant pain. Suddenly, anything—no, *everything*—felt possible.

Each month, I would have a flare-up around my lady time, and fear would grip me, reminding me of how life used to be pain 24/7. The weeks of low or no pain gave me hope and made me realize how badly I wanted to be totally healthy, and how afraid I was it wouldn't work. That fear motivated me to push on.

It wasn't an easy process. My healing took time and patience. My sleeping schedule was random from years of not sleeping. I had to sleep-train like a child and relearn how to get a full night's rest. I used meditation tapes to still my mind. I appreciated the way a forty-five-minute nap without pain could heal. (Sometimes it's the little things.)

I also had to be patient reentering my daily activities. As my pain-free hours became more frequent, I was excited about the prospect of "doing stuff" again. I wanted to get outside, walk my dogs. However, after just a block, I'd have to hobble back and lie down as if I'd run a marathon.

Seeing Is Believing

I wasn't the only one who got better on this crazy diet. I got to see its effect close-up after sharing it with my then-boss.

When I interviewed for the job with him and his partners, I decided transparency was the best policy. I told them I was good at my job, but very sick, and would most likely work from home a lot; they really shouldn't hire me. However, I promised that when I had "good days" I would be in and giving it my all. They hired me on the spot. Go figure.

My boss was tall, dynamic, a strict vegetarian. His lifestyle was the definition of "healthy." I found out later that he had struggled with Crohn's disease years earlier, and had a piece of his intestines removed. The operation was supposed to fix him; instead, it gave him a whole new level of gut sensitivity, exacerbating the effects of Crohn's. Not only had the operation cut out a portion of his body's system for absorbing nutrients, but he felt the effects of scar tissue that had resulted from the surgery. While we were working together, he had a massive "flare," and at 6′ 6″ tall, he dropped to 190 pounds in a blink of an eye. Where I was filled with intense pain and was a "shitter" (if you will), he was a "bleeder." His doctor was advocating for removing his colon altogether.

When I started following Karen's diet, I sat down and

chatted about it with him over lunch. "Look, I know it may appear that I'm a crazy hippie doing this crazy diet, and I don't know if it's going to work," I told him. "But it's my last stop before I agree to endless meds and, most likely, multiple surgeries. I don't expect you to try it, but I wanted to let you know, in case you wanted to check it out."

He read Karen's book and also got the feeling I had—"this is so crazy, it just might work." He decided to give the diet a try, and put off the surgery his doctor recommended. This choice was controversial for the people in his life. His family wasn't convinced; they were scared for his health. His mother even called me to get the lowdown on the diet I'd recommended to her son. Late at night, while I walked the halls of my small house, I worried that I might be killing my boss with my alternative approach to healing.

To my surprise, despite being technically in worse shape than me, he got better before I did. Within six months of starting Karen's diet, he was feeling well, gaining weight, eating with vigor, and not on any medication, on his way to living a normal life. I was overjoyed...not to mention envious AF.

We became Crohn's buddies, talked constantly on the phone, providing emotional support to each other, sharing tips on implementing our weird but effective diet.

Other people would have overheard us and said, "You guys are fucking crazy." Believe me, we knew how crazy we sounded, but we were so excited to have a diet that worked and a friend who understood. Over those months of healing and working together, we formed a bond that felt unbreakable. Definitely my soul brother.

Looking back, I wonder if some cosmic force brought me into that company. It was priceless to have a friend on the journey I was taking. I realized what an amazing gift it is to have someone with whom you can speak openly about what you're going through. It was just as healing as the diet itself.

Most people suffering from an autoimmune disorder don't know anyone who can share their experience. Illness often feels like a burden. Those who know other sufferers often still feel alone, because everyone's symptoms manifest differently. Those who try to heal naturally, instead of taking drugs or choosing surgery, often feel isolated. Being able to reach out and talk to someone can make all the difference in moving forward on your healing journey.

Feeling Good Does Not Make You Fine

Most people, unless they're born with an ailment, live on their own terms, not on their body's terms. They don't consider their body's need for sleep, nutritious food, or a healthy lifestyle.

For most of my adult life, I thought if I felt good, and as long as I was slender, things were fine. I was healthy, right? I had no idea that, behind the scenes, my body was constantly making up for my lack of nutrients, stealing from Peter to pay Paul, neutralizing the chemicals I ingested in my foods and through my beauty products and the crap I put on my skin. I had no idea that my homeostasis was a precarious balance, until I was unable to stand up and scramble eggs for my kids, take them for a hike, or sit in an auditorium while they performed in their school play.

I regret that it took getting sick (and not knowing whether I would ever get better) for me to shift my lazy, appearance-based mentality around health, and stop letting my asshole taste buds make all my decisions for me.

It wasn't until I was a shattered pile of human flesh on the floor in the kitchen at night, so hungry but unable to eat, dehydrated yet nauseous at the sight of water, down to skin and bone because my body had been feeding off its own tissue, that I clearly saw the damage of letting my taste buds run my life.

I'm not a particularly religious person, but I remember,

in that moment, saying to God, the universe, or all that is, *Take my life or let me get better, because I can't do this. This isn't living. Every day, my body is just dying a little bit more. If I do get better, I promise I will find a way to give back.*

(Hey, God? This book is my start in that direction.)

I didn't know I would get better, or what giving back would look like. I just knew that's what it had to be. Once I was well, I would help other people heal.

You're Already On Your Way

It took time to heal, but as soon as I did, I left my amazing job to take some time off, enjoy my newfound health and my family, and take a moment to contemplate the next chapter of my life. In that time, I remembered the promise I'd made to help others, and signed up for a health coaching course. I wanted to start helping people now.

Furthermore, I wanted to help not just people with autoimmune issues, but all kinds of people. I wanted to become an advocate for preventative medicine. After all, it's super hard (and scary) to heal once you are sick. It's so much better and easier to live healthily.

These days, I love being there for others, whether they are

suffering the way I used to, or just in need of some health support. Whether you need a cheerleader, a shoulder to cry on, or a voice of reason when everyone around you is telling you to just take the drugs, I'm here to listen, empathize, encourage, and serve as living proof that healing is possible. When we're tackling the mountains in this journey toward health, we all need someone who has been down a similar road and can help cheer us on.

I remember how it feels to think things can't get worse, and then wake up the next day to find they have. I'm here to remind you why it's such an amazing gift to go through this healing process for your body, and how priceless it will be when you make it through to the other side. When you're so sick and tired of being sick and tired that you're ready to explode, I'm here to say, "Ya, I know, this sucks, but guess what? After you go through this part of your life, you get to have it back again. You won't be missing part of your intestines. You won't be on medications that have all these side effects. And if you flare, you can always go back to step one—I did it many times before I went into total remission. Surrender to the journey. You can do this."

I know it takes work to turn things around. That's why I've written this book sharing my story. I want to inspire you and give you some hope that although natural healing takes time, effort, and great commitment, hopefully my story will encourage you to push you through the final mile to wellness.

Wherever you are on your health journey, you're great, and you're going to be even greater. It's our journey that makes us who we are and shows us what we are made of. And you, my friend, are made of greatness.

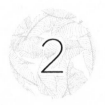

Killing Me Not
So Softly

· · · · · · ·

Crohn's caught me at a time when my life was very full.
I had two young daughters. I was a partner in an artist
management company in the ad biz. I was recently remar-
ried—we were practically still newlyweds, married only
a year. My life was in full swing.

For the past eight months, I'd been experiencing "stomach issues" like never before—upset stomach, diarrhea,
food sensitivities, the whole nine. I kept insisting it had
to be something I ate. I'd had these issues before and
they'd gone away after a day or two. But this time, they
were not only hanging around a lot longer, but hurting a
lot more. I couldn't simply sleep off the pain or nurse my
upset stomach with a heating pad.

There were new issues showing up, too. Smells bothered me on a cellular level. I couldn't come in the kitchen when food was cooking. I cleared all scented products from the house entirely. I couldn't be around people wearing perfume. All it took was a whiff to trigger my nausea. I also started dropping weight at an alarming rate.

Those symptoms—cramping pain, diarrhea, intense nausea—built up, side by side, until I couldn't ignore them anymore. I had to see a doctor.

Going the "Natural" Route

My parents hated the entire medical world and went to great lengths to keep us far from a doctor's office. My siblings and I were born at home and raised on home remedies. However, my father was firm in his belief that there were "healers" in the world—people who, in addition to their medical training, had an intuitive understanding of the human body and were gifted in helping the body naturally overcome disease and pain.

With that in mind, I've always had a real love and respect for doctors. Long before my disease showed up, if I heard a general practitioner or specialist recommended enthusiastically from a friend, I would make a note and sometimes even book an appointment to just get a "tune-up." I was fascinated by what they did and learning about what made their patients passionate about them. One might say this was some interesting foreshadowing going on.

At my daughters' preschool, I met a fellow parent and renowned Chinese medicine doctor. People raved about him so much that I immediately booked a session for a tune-up. When the constant pain and weight loss began setting off my alarm bells, he was one of the first people I went to. After a few weeks of seeing him on a regular basis and my symptoms getting worse, he suggested I see a gastroenterologist he knew and respected. This was the moment when I realized that shit must be more serious than I thought.

Right from the start, I told this GI that I wanted to heal naturally. To him, I must have seemed crazy. Here I was in his office, skinny and shaking with pain, yet seeking no immediate reprieve. I know a lot of people in my life couldn't understand why I didn't take the drugs being offered to me by my doctors. If nothing else, they said, I should relieve myself of the constant pain undermining my life in every possible way. I was losing weight. I had arthritis in my hands and my joints. My skin started getting rashes. My hair was falling out in handfuls. I had sores everywhere, from mouth to tail. The weight of my husband's hand was more than I could tolerate.

Needless to say, it was not a super sexy time in my life.

Oh, and did I mention the amount of pain I was in? Fuuuuuck.

I've given birth without an epidural twice in my life, and the pain of Crohn's disease was far worse than that. Everything caused me intense pain, and when I ate I could feel every inch of it moving through my digestive tract like a Brillo pad. Often, it sent me running to the bathroom in emergency mode to what I coined "painting the walls." There were many times when I had to decide between vomiting or shitting on the floor. (I chalk this confusion up to extreme pain—in my right mind, I definitely know what goes where.)

I was so nauseous and in so much pain, I could barely get anything past my lips. The inflammation in my ilium was so fucking intense, making it impossible to absorb nutrients from the little food I was able to get down. And because I couldn't digest or eliminate food properly, I couldn't detoxify. I also couldn't regulate my emotions, because my gut wasn't manufacturing hormones the way it's supposed to. In the middle of talking or listening, I would start sobbing uncontrollably. The pain and the hopelessness of the scenario would just hit me like a ton of bricks. I needed help, and I needed it now.

Did I Want to Be Sick?

Being an open-minded kind of gal, I visited a kinesiology expert who came recommended by a good friend. This lady was convinced my problem was caused by a parasite, maybe one I'd picked up in my travels abroad. She used an esoteric form of diagnosis called "muscle testing" that was popular in Los Angeles—it uses your body's reflexive responses to determine what nutrients you're lacking. I took the vitamins and supplements she gave me, and for a little while, they seemed to be helping. But soon I had nosedived again. When I told her this, she responded by saying something I'd never thought of:

"You want to be sick."

At first, I didn't know how to respond. I even wondered if she was right. I told my husband what she'd said, and he thought I should explore the possibility just to rule it out. How we feel about ourselves and our health is powerful and important to reflect on.

I reflected as hard as I could, wondering if there was something in me that secretly wanted to be sick. I didn't have an easy childhood or a close relationship with my parents. But after a deep inquiry, all I could come up with was my powerful will to live. I had run away from home in search of a better life for myself. That's not something a person who wants to be sick does. At this point in my life, I had worked hard to create a happy life for myself. I had awesome kids, a sweet job, a groovy husband, all of which I loved. I wanted to keep enjoying my life at full blast until I was ninety years old.

The results of reflection were in: I genuinely wanted to be better. Fuck that kinesiologist with her "you want to be sick" bullshit. I ditched her fast and hard and continued on my healing journey.

Looking For Help

As my stomach issues worsened, I looked for a doctor who could help me. I wouldn't just go in for a check-up; I'd follow up with lots of emails, asking all kinds of questions. I visited several doctors at the most reputable healthcare centers in Los Angeles—everywhere from Cedar Sinai to UCLA. I wanted someone I could trust, someone who wouldn't just write me a prescription or insist on surgery. I needed a partner in healing. I needed a hero.

Each time I would arrive at a doctor's appointment, explain my symptoms and my history, and listen to them tell me all the things it could be (which by that time I already knew). Then, the tests would start. All of them drew blood, and everything always came back the same—from a blood test perspective, I was healthy. (Somehow that small fact gave me amazing hope.)

They'd run the blood tests again and again. Then they'd move on to checking my ankles. I found out later this was to test my ability to absorb protein—apparently, the ankles swell when your body isn't taking in protein properly. I did breath tests for an overgrowth of H. pylori bacteria and stool tests for parasites.

At one point, one of the GIs I saw suggested there *could* be a parasite inside me that they didn't have a test for. This seemed like an easy fix—I was eager for anything that sounded like an explanation, so I got behind this diagnosis. However, I wasn't thrilled about his solution: a round of heavy duty, carpet-bomb-your-entire-system antibiotics to clear out the possible mystery parasite. I was desperate for some relief, some possible solution to my pain, and I agreed to do the antibiotics. BAD IDEA.

Not only did the antibiotics not work, but my health took an even deeper nosedive. (I didn't even know that was possible. Son of a bitch.) By taking the antibiotics, I'd killed off all the beneficial bacteria in my system working overtime to fight off inflammation and disease in my gut. Without any equilibrium inside my gut, my body rejected food entirely. I was worse off than before. Can you imagine? Yeah, me neither; I still try to block that shit out.

This was a horrendous part of the journey for me. Between nonstop doctor visits, lab work, and special diets, these were the most expensive years I'd ever lived. Even worse was how these doctors looked at me when I said I wanted to heal naturally, especially once they knew I'd already consulted several great GIs in town. "What are you looking for?" they were saying to me, in so many words. "This is the protocol. These doctors that you're seeing are good— we're all going to back each other up and say this is the only path you can go down."

I would leave the appointment sobbing, wanting to drive my car right into the sea, pedal to the metal. I felt so hopeless, so defeated at the lack of options available to me. Then, I would look at the alternative to continuing my path—going on drugs that had the potential to give me cancer, letting them cut out a piece of my intestines—and I would think, *No. As soon as I let them cut me open, I'm changing my body forever*. So I stayed with the devils I knew: pain and agony.

I understand for some people, there is no other option but surgery. We all have our own personal breaking point. For some people, that point ends in saying, "Cut that shit out and let's cover it up; just make it go away so I can get back to living." I can definitely respect that feeling, but for me, that just wasn't the right choice. Instead, I buckled down and summoned a power I didn't know I had.

Our intestines absorb the majority of our nutrients. I believe we have them at a certain length for a reason. Our bodies were made perfect—every inch of us is there for a purpose. As far as it's in my power, I'm going to keep it as nature intended.

In the dark of night, I often felt hopeless and desperate, wondering if I had missed the exit, if I was just being stubborn. And then I would watch the sun rise, and feel a sense of hope fill my aching body as I embarked on another day of trying to find the needle in the haystack.

My Hippie Roots

I should explain why I was so determined not to go on medication or antibiotics.

I was raised by the quintessential California hippies. One of eight kids born at home in Big Sur, raised in a household as "all-natural" as you can get. My parents were very spiritual, intentionally connected to the earth. We were dirt poor, but rich with knowledge and appreciation. My father was in so many ways ahead of his time. He raised us to believe that your food becomes your body, and your body becomes part of the spirit of the food you're eating. My parents didn't believe in traditional medicine. Instead, we lived as close to the earth as possible, living healthy, whole lives, respecting our bodies and the food we put into them. When I left home, my father told me, "If you have the choice, between a nourishing meal and a pair of shoes, pick the wholesome meal." Yeah, right. Eye roll. Gonna get me some sweet-ass shoes.

I'd come a long way since then, but those principles stayed with me. Even though I'd spent my late teens and twenties veering off the healthy path my parents taught me, when I found myself getting sick, I was determined not to make myself sicker through invasive procedures or pharmaceutical medication if at all possible. The hippie within was suddenly very much awake beneath my somewhat normal exterior.

The doctors blew my mind when they told me my immune system was attacking my body. (Say *what?*) For that reason, they recommended drugs like 6-MP, Remicade, and Humira, all of which are designed to suppress the immune system. To me, that didn't sit right. Why would my immune system attack me? That doesn't make sense. My immune system is there to protect me. If I suppress it, then I'm laying myself open to all sorts of attacks from the outside. Right?

To me, that was a scarier proposition than the current pain I was in. Honestly, I wasn't sure my frail body could handle an invasive surgery. Beyond that, my intuition told me I didn't need this stuff. If it came to a last resort, then I might consider surgery or immune suppressant drugs. My commitment to life, to surviving for the sake of my daughters and my husband, gave me the assurance I wouldn't get to a point where there was no turning back; but I wasn't going there until I'd searched the earth far and wide for somebody who understood why my body was giving the appearance of attacking me. I needed a healer, someone who understood the body on a holistic level and believed it could heal.

You could call it stubbornness, or maybe even stupidity. You could call it dedication. You could call it blind hope. At this point, I think of it as just being a real belief in my body's ability and desire to heal. I knew if I could find the "cause" and remove it, then I could heal. Easier said than done.

It made perfect sense to me that my entire body would be sick when the intestines were sick. The idea that they could cut out the intestines, and suddenly my illness would vanish, didn't make sense to me. It sounded like playing "whack-a-mole" with your health—as soon as you cut out one problem area, the issue is going to pop up in another area. I wasn't ready to sign up for a life of ongoing surgery or medication.

At one point, my general practitioner did something surprising: he prescribed me marijuana. As someone who grew up in a community where smoking weed was the norm, you might think I would have been a lot more open to this idea. However, I had two young daughters and felt strange about bringing it into our home at that time.

My GP was appropriately laid-back on this topic. "You can't sleep, you can't eat, and you're in constant pain," he pointed out. "I can give you five different prescriptions to help with those things, or you can try just this one. I've never prescribed this to anyone in my twenty-something years of being in practice, but I know you want to heal as naturally as possible. Well, this is as natural as it gets." He winked as he handed me the prescription. "At least you'll be able to eat."

I took the prescription, not missing the irony that my hippie upbringing was coming back full circle. Still, I held onto the prescription for three months before I had it filled. My husband demanded it. The lady at the dispensary looked at my prescription and said, "Oh, you have Crohn's. We get a lot of people with Crohn's."

After I explained my symptoms—pain and nausea—she gave me a couple of vials of CBD flower. CBD is a different chemical compound from THC, which creates the mind-altering high most people associate with marijuana. She also handed me some potent THC flower; she said it would help with the pain. Yep, good shit—highly recommend.

While this book is mainly about the healing diet I used to overcome Crohn's, I have to point out that there were several things that made that diet accessible to me. After all, you need to actually get the food past your lips for the diet to make a difference. In this regard, weed helped me so much. Once I started the diet, it took a full year (plus change) for me to go into remission from Crohn's. There were a lot of days where I needed something to get past the nausea and pain long enough to eat the food that would help heal me. Once the nausea abated, I could eat because, the munchies! Smoking also allowed me to sleep through some of the pain. Sometimes I toked up at least ten times in a single day, and not just for fun, although I won't lie: the state it put me in really helped my sense of humor. It didn't take the pain away, but it changed my relationship to the pain. Somehow the pain was further away, not up in my face trying to pick a fight.

I never thought as a parent I'd be smoking weed in my own home. However, at this point in my journey, I would try just about anything that would provide some natural pain relief, alleviate the nausea, and give me back a few winks. I might have binge-watched Ren and Stimpy in my altered state. Knowing that sleep is necessary for our bodies to heal and regenerate from the wear and tear of a given day, sleeping and eating became my top priorities. When you have a serious internal problem, it's twice as crucial and devastating when sleep eludes you. I would walk the halls of my little bungalow for years, like a ghost, half sobbing, half screaming, knowing every minute I wasn't sleeping was a minute my body wasn't healing. If I was lucky, I'd pass out from sheer exhaustion for twenty to thirty minutes. It may not sound like much, but for me, these short bouts of sleep were pure bliss.

No Good Options

While I was working with my Chinese medicine doctor, he said that it was important we give a name to the mysterious issue ravaging my health. However, I found myself unwilling to do this. It felt like there was something easier, or less scary, about keeping it mysterious. For some reason, naming the disease gave it too much power in my mind. I was afraid if I identified it, it would own me for the rest of my life.

Of course, doctors are all about naming the disease. Along with the suggestion of parasites, infections, and IBS, the possibility of Crohn's disease was brought up more than once by the doctors I saw.

When I'd ask them how we could heal it, they'd tell me there wasn't anything to heal it. Crohn's, they said, is something you just have to manage for the rest of your life. "You can go gluten-free," one of them said. "That seems to help people with Crohn's." It was like they viewed disease as being disconnected from the body.

All the research out there was hopeless, indicating a life-long dedication to managing symptoms. I wasn't ready to surrender to that life sentence. I was determined to explore every possible option to know without a shadow of a doubt that was the only way.

But it didn't matter, I told myself, because I didn't fit the profile for Crohn's disease. It didn't run in my family. My blood work was still okay, showing no signs of inflammation. So the search for a cure went on, while the disease remained unnamed.

Meanwhile, I was getting sicker and sicker, with no good reason why. I've since learned one of the problems with Crohn's is that it shows up differently for everybody. That's how the GI finally convinced me I needed to do an endoscopy (stomach camera) and a colonoscopy (butt camera).

I agreed to the procedures, even though I was afraid of being put under. Yeah, I know; laugh at me. I can withstand horrendous pain, but suggest putting me under and I become a big baby. To be honest, I wasn't sure my body could handle the procedure. But as we were running out of options, I gave in. Snake the drain, homeboy.

In the end, the procedures turned out to be a mixed blessing. They revealed my stomach was fine, but the small intestine was entirely inflamed and closed for business. In other words, I pretty much had a classic presentation for severe Crohn's disease.

And you know what? Once we gave it a name, I felt a sense of power. Instead of feeling like my painful, sick condition was taking hold of my life, I felt like I could suddenly make this illness my bitch. That renewed my motivation and hope for finding a way to remove it.

I knew it would be like finding a needle in a haystack. The doctors I'd talked to were all convinced that Crohn's wasn't a matter of healing, but managing. Prescription drugs, interventions, and surgery came up again and again.

But now that I knew what was wrong, I was more determined than ever not to cut it out and cover it up. If anything, that option put the fear of God into me—I knew that's where I would end up, if I didn't find the answer. That was not a place I wanted to be, playing "whack-a-mole" with my health.

Learning to Value My Gift

I came to accept that I didn't "get" Crohn's by accident. It was the end of a long, convoluted path I'd been walking my entire adulthood without realizing it. Sure, my genes might have given me a sensitivity, but my reckless lifestyle choices pulled the stupid trigger.

We've all heard it said a million times, but it's true: *You are what you eat.* I heard that from my parents all my life; to be honest, part of me hated having to acknowledge it was true.

The time I spent battling Crohn's was instrumental, in many ways. Before that time, I was like any regular asshole. I ran myself ragged, worked crazy hours without enough sleep, and went out drinking several nights in a row. I made choices based on what I wanted, versus what was best for me. I didn't consider my body or the long-term effects my choices could have on it. If my jeans fit, I considered myself healthy. Um, hello? Disconnect, anyone? Health is not skin deep.

Being chronically ill was like having a mirror shoved in my face: *Wake up! This is your body! This is the vehicle that allows you to travel the world, achieve your dreams, watch your children grow up, meet your grandchildren...if you take care of it.*

When that moment came, I felt guilty. I felt like I had disrespected the greatest gift we have as humans. The body is what lets us do everything that gives us the most joy: run, jump, skip, play ball, pet our dogs, make sexy time with those we love. It was the one thing I never considered while making choices in my life.

Humans' greatest threat used to be something big and scary killing them. Today, it's us killing ourselves with the shit we mindlessly shove into our faces. The advances we have made as a species create a disconnect with *what* we are. We're made of food—proteins, fats, carbohydrates. We're creating stuff for ourselves to eat—stuff that tastes like food, but isn't food. Meanwhile, we're lacing real food with man-made chemicals that have nothing to do with nature. Chemicals that keep bugs away from crops; chemicals that speed up or slow down the ripening process while our produce travels hundreds of miles to the grocery store; chemicals that keep dead food alive, like zombies, on the shelf for weeks.

Scientists are speculating that people are moving toward the shortest lifespans they've had in a long time, because of the illness created in recent decades. You can trace that trend of disease back to environmental toxicity, especially within the food chain. Yet we still argue whether organic produce is worth the extra money.

Let's pause for a minute so you can ask yourself this question: How much *is* good health and longevity worth? I can tell you firsthand that disease is a lot more expensive and harder to come back from than buying organic, local, healthful foods in the first place.

When I was a kid, you seldom heard of cancer. Now, I feel like every person I know is friends with somebody who has cancer, if they haven't experienced cancer themselves. If that's not a reason to look in the mirror and ask yourself some serious questions about what you're putting in and on your body, I don't know what is.

To get ourselves back on a path to health and longevity, we must intervene assertively. We can't assume our doctors are the experts and everything they say is best. As I said before, I think doctors are great in certain situations, and I have a huge respect for what they do, but your doctor will never be the same advocate for your health that you can be. You are the one putting food in your mouth and stuff on your skin. These are the choices that build a healthy body, or a diseased body. These are the choices that support your body's ability to protect itself and flourish.

Ultimately, your body is your vehicle through this world. You must stay connected to it if you want to be healthy. If you find yourself sick, you should consider whether it's necessary to "overhaul the engine," or whether you're better off making a few essential tweaks to your food and lifestyle choices.

A NOTE TO THE HEALTHY PEOPLE

This book isn't only for people actively struggling with Crohn's. If you're a healthy person, my hope is to inspire you to contemplate what health means to you. Maybe at a deeper level than you may have considered before.

I'm a person who loves life, and my guess is that you do, too. No matter what the state of your health looks like now, my hope is that this book encourages you in your journey. No matter what issues you deal with, whether they're occasional or chronic, your body has the amazing ability to heal itself, albeit maybe not overnight. A broken body, like a broken heart, takes time to heal. With some dedication and perseverance, you can experience the priceless gift of a life lived fully and well.

I had people in my life so worried for me, thinking I'd get sick beyond the point of turning back, or my inflammation would get so bad something would rupture and I'd die. They'd plead with me to "try" the drugs, just for a "little while" to see if it helped.

I understood why they said that. It made sense on paper. Toward the end, I felt so crazy—both from the pain and the frustration of searching for a solution—I wondered if they were right. It may sound crazy to you. Why not take the drugs temporarily and get some relief? Why not trust the best doctors in the field?

I had this lingering feeling I couldn't shake. I felt that there was something about the pain I could understand. If I kept looking, I would find the healing answer to my disease question.

Despite all the pain and frustration, there was a rock-solid assurance underneath it all that, far from attacking me, my body was trying to tell me something. I couldn't believe it would attack me for no reason. The human organism is incredibly intelligent in the way it's built to protect us. My job was to hear and interpret it, not to stifle its message by cutting it out through surgery or covering it up with drugs.

If I effectively stuffed a sock in my body's mouth, I

wouldn't "hear" it anymore, but then where would I be? Who would I be?

Healing Your Body Starts with Hearing Your Body

If you're like me, you've taken your body for granted most of your life. When it sends you messages through pain and illness, it's confusing and alarming. The easiest way to deal with these feelings is to take an Advil and move on, right?

In contrast, learning to understand your body is like learning to speak another language. In many ways, it's like being a parent of a toddler who knows what they want to say to you, but can't form the words—you're constantly having to ask questions and eliminate what they're not saying.

My journey through Crohn's was a series of finding out what *wasn't* the right answer. I tried one thing after another, looking for the help my body needed. Everything I thought would work failed me.

The turning point came when I stopped assuming what worked for others would work for me. I had to allow this to become an individual journey of discovering my body and realizing it was more than I thought it was.

What's interesting about this diet—which I'll be taking you through in the next chapter—is that it has worked for many different people, not just people with Crohn's. I've watched it heal people with ulcerative colitis, Hashimoto's disease, even people who have had multiple surgeries. It's not dependent on your symptoms. The success of this diet is in its ability to locate and pull out the stinger causing your issues in the first place. It presumes your body knows what it's telling you—far from attacking you, it's trying to get your attention about something wrong. This diet is the only one I've found that allows you to work with your body and support it gently while it heals itself. Inflammation is actually the body trying to protect itself so it can heal. AMAZING.

Everything out there for Crohn's disease is about symptom management. It was disheartening that nobody offered hope I could heal. I believe autoimmune disorders result from the body's inability to eliminate toxic man-made waste. Real relief only comes when you can find what's causing that core issue and remove it.

Ultimately, *you* get to decide what's right for your body. If you feel surgery is right for you, this book isn't about convincing you otherwise. It is, however, meant to convince you that you are made of what you eat. If you eat in such a way that you're aiding your body and giving it the proper nutrients so it can detox and heal properly, then you, too, can find health again. There is, indeed, another option. I want you to live a life of radiant health, not on the edge wondering when the next flare will pull you away from the life you love. There's no reason to let pain and suffering bench you on the sidelines while others live the dream.

You deserve to live life to the fullest. Don't let anyone or anything convince you otherwise.

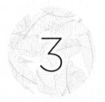

The Problem Behind the Problem of Crohn's

. . . .

We all have that person in our life—maybe it's your friend, your relative, or your spouse—who can eat whatever they want and seems to always have tons of energy, good health, great skin, and no digestive trouble at all. You look at them and think, "A 'normal' diet works for them—it should work the same for me." We ignore what our bodies are telling us because we don't want to take the time to reform our habits of eating whatever we want, whenever we want, even if we know from experience that eating like "everybody else" does not work out well for us.

I was like this, too. I cared more about how I looked than about what the food I ate was doing in my body. I worked out like crazy, I ate some salads, I drank smoothies and juice instead of soda—I thought that was healthy enough.

When I'd be on the road for my advertising job, I would take clients out and get people hammered. I would tell myself that it was fine—I wasn't getting too drunk, I was "spacing it out" all night. But the reality was that I was still overindulging in everything. I wasn't eating consciously; I was consuming whatever came my way. I was living while my body was dying.

Even when I did make healthy choices, it wasn't out of a desire to protect my health. If I avoided M&Ms, it wasn't because they are covered in Yellow #5 and Yellow #6; it was because I didn't want that extra pound or two preventing me from fitting into my wardrobe. It wasn't about health, it was about appearance. My relationship to health was skin deep.

Now, of course, I understand that thin doesn't mean healthy. As a result, I don't always consider people lucky when they can eat whatever they want.

Some people's bodies seem to handle toxicity very well, especially the kind that comes from external sources like immunization, food additives, medication, environmental toxins, etc. When I meet people like this, I think, "You're a unicorn. You're not even human." My particular physical makeup happens to be one that doesn't tolerate toxicity well. That's why I'm not holding my body to the standard set by unicorns. Instead, I'm going to treat it with the care it deserves.

I don't feel deprived because my body refuses to put up with toxicity. I feel like I'm the lucky one for knowing what my body needs to stay healthy. After all, it's the only one I'm going to get.

Your Body Is Smarter Than You Give It Credit For

All the doctors I saw described Crohn's disease as "my body attacking itself." That never made sense to me—it still doesn't. Why would the body attack itself?

I think a more accurate description is that Crohn's is a state of inflammation caused by the body not being able to detoxify properly. Now, I'm just a person—I'm not a doctor or a scientist. But I'm basing this description on the fact that this Desperation Diet works on people with Crohn's because it helps the body detoxify while replenishing all the vitamins, minerals, and essential proteins needed to maintain a healthy body.

The fact is that a lot of the elements that have been labeled safe or harmless by scientists are not properly tested and proven over the long haul. It's still debatable whether our bodies can handle it or not. Think of it this way: if one person pees in the pool, it's not going to change the pH balance of the entire pool, but if everybody does it every day, pretty soon that pool is going to be a pretty different environment. It's the same idea with your body. It's true that one crappy meal isn't going to send your body into a toxic tailspin. But when factory-farmed, preservative-laced food is the foundation of your diet, guess what? You've got a "too much pee in the pool" situation.

Here's a slightly less icky way to think about it:

If you build a house with quality materials, you have a house that has the potential to last forever. If you build a house with cheap materials, that house is going to start falling down at some point. That's the whole premise behind eating for longevity of health, and I think it makes a lot of damn sense, don't you?

It couldn't be more fitting that the acronym for "standard American diet" is SAD. It's setting people up to live in a body that doesn't stay healthy and whole throughout their lives. It's not going to withstand the test of time—it's going to fall apart. When it starts to deteriorate, we don't take that as a sign that it's time to make changes. Instead, we inject ourselves with all kinds of stuff, or we pop pills as if there is no consequence.

Unless you're eating a diet that's high in organic produce, healthy fat, and grass-fed meats or vegetable protein, along with soluble fiber, your body most likely isn't getting rid of the toxins it takes in. If your bile doesn't have something to bind to, something that can transport it out from the body, then those foreign toxins are going to keep rotating through the body. Eventually, all that toxicity will show up in the form of one disease or another.

The truth is that our bodies are incredibly smart. They don't just attack themselves for no reason. If anything, they are so determined to live that they refuse to go down quietly. If you're in the midst of an autoimmune illness, it means your body is sending up every distress signal it can find, just to get your attention that something in your lifestyle needs to change. Wake up and listen!

Let's Talk About Bile

It's time for some down-and-dirty talk about the body's garbage system. Ready?

It starts with the liver and a digestive fluid it makes called bile. Bile is used to break down/convert/neutralize everything that comes into our bodies—the food we eat, the stuff we spread on our skin, the air we breathe, the water we drink, etc. Bile helps convert vitamins and minerals into usable forms, and does its best to neutralize all those delicious toxins we've absorbed.

The liver manufactures bile and sends it to the gallbladder, where it's stored until a meal is eaten. When we eat, the gallbladder releases a significant amount of the bile into the first part of our small intestine (known as the duodenum). That's where bile begins to break down the food we've consumed.

Next, the bile travels from the duodenum to the jejunum, where most of the nutrients (the stuff our bodies can actually use) are absorbed. After that absorption process, all that's left in the bile are toxins and chemicals: the body's garbage.

From there, the bile travels to the ileum. At that point, something very significant happens. If there is soluble fiber available, bile will bind to it and be shuttled out of the body in the form of—you guessed it—poop.

But if there isn't sufficient soluble fiber, the bile will be absorbed into the terminal part of the ileum and be returned to the liver, so that it can be used again for another round of garbage collection.

Now, in a healthy body, there will be plenty of soluble fiber and a minimum of garbage to get rid of. In this scenario, the bile recycling system works great, and it's a very efficient use of the body's resources.

But in a modern American body, where there's an excess of toxins and a minimal amount of soluble fiber, you end up with a lot of garbage-filled liquid being circulated throughout the body, over and over. In fact, about 99 percent of what should be excreted in the bile ends up being reabsorbed into the body. The more this happens, the more irritation builds up, until you're looking at full-blown inflammation.

This whole bile recycling system is why Crohn's disease tends to present at the ileocecal valve, the spot where the ileum meets the large intestine. That's where the uptake of bile happens, and it's where the bile should start the process of being pooped out. But if the bile hasn't created a bond with soluble fiber somewhere along the way, the ileocecal valve is where the body reroutes the bile (along with all the garbage it's carrying) back through the system into the liver for storage, until the next time it's needed.

It's important to understand that bile is made up of water,

minerals, neutralized toxins, and cholesterol (fat). One of the most popular healing diets at the time I was getting really sick was the paleo diet, which centered on drinking bone broth and consuming a lot of healthy fats. For some people, this diet had amazing results. I couldn't understand why I wasn't getting better on it, too.

At the time, I didn't know the simple fact that when you eat fat, even healthy fat, your body has to produce more bile to break it down. More bile in my body just equaled more pain and suffering. For a person like me with an inflamed gut, consuming fat in any form was like pouring battery acid down my throat.

That's why, when I started Karen's diet, I avoided all forms of dietary fat for a bit. No olive oil, no butter, nothing. Anything I cooked had to be cooked in a dry pan. When I started eating meat, it had to be super lean. I had to alleviate some of the bile production in order to get rid of what was already there, and give my body an opportunity to heal.

Different Presentations of Crohn's

Crohn's disease is a sneaky SOB because it shows up differently for different people. As I mentioned earlier, my boss was a bleeder. Some people have fistulas (nasty little pockets of pus inside the body), rashes, hemorrhoids, sores everywhere. The one consistent symptom is constant diarrhea. I'm not talking about once a day—I mean more like twenty times per day.

I was really fascinated to find out that for some people, Crohn's disease presents little to no pain. They can be having diarrhea all day, but there's no blood or pain to send them running to the doctor.

My GI, Dr. T., told me that he preferred the patient who experienced pain with Crohn's disease, versus the person who has no pain presentation. If the person chose to ignore the diarrhea, they can go their entire lives or as long as they can without knowing that it's a problem.

Personally, I had very little bleeding, but I did get heavy-duty pain. I was so bloated that my stomach looked like I was in my first trimester of pregnancy, and I farted a ton. Needless to say, it was not a time in my life when I felt super sexy.

At my weakest, I could no longer wear normal workout shoes, and had to hit the shoe store looking for a lighter solution. They looked at me sideways when I explained my situation, and brought out those five-toe shoes to me. I thought they looked ridiculous, but then I put them on, and I was like, "Oh my God, they're so light. I can walk in them." The five-toe shoes allowed me to actually walk a block further before turning back. It wasn't long before I started to really love those shoes—after all, they allowed me to get outside again.

As I got strong and stronger, I still continued to wear those five-toe shoes. I got used to them and the funny looks I got. Recently, I was walking the dog when a young woman walked towards us from the opposite direction. As she passed me, she looked at my shoes and smirked, and I don't know why but I turned around to look at her as we passed each other. Her back was to me by that point, and I saw that she was wearing a Hello Kitty backpack. I'll admit it—I smirked. If a grown woman is out there wearing a Hello Kitty backpack, I'm going to go ahead and feel pretty good about my five-toe shoes.

The more inflamed my gut became, the less I could eat, and my muscles began to break down. My gums bled, I lost hair, and my skin let off a really weird smell. The best way I can describe it is the way someone smells when they've been in the hospital a long time. I'd take a shower and still smell sick when I got out. I stopped using any kind of scented soap or lotion—everything hurt to smell.

Crohn's never quit showing up in unexpected places. I can remember going for a dental cleaning, and the technician started lecturing me about the excessive bleeding and tartar they'd found on my teeth. I had to explain to them that my dental habits hadn't changed—I had a chronic bowel disease. (I don't think they made the connection.)

It all goes to show that the body really is one organism. You don't just get sick in one part of your body. When one thing isn't working, the entire body isn't working. Inflammation is like a wildfire, destroying everything in its path.

Because Crohn's can look any number of different ways, it's pretty common that a treatment that works for one person will do little or nothing for someone else.

Most doctors, if they're honest, will admit that they only have part of the picture when it comes to Crohn's. They don't have all the answers. If they did, they could say, "Okay, these are the diets that work for people. Try these diets first and if none of them work, then let's try immune suppressants. If that doesn't work, we can cut it out as a last resort."

The fact that they immediately go to a fistful of meds and start the conversation of cutting it out and covering it up was, for me, a red flag. My journey made me realize that it's much easier to keep a healthy person "healthy" than it is to dig a person out of the bottom of the barrel, so to speak.

Even though I've found that the Desperation Diet has a powerful healing impact on everyone I've coached, I still leave a lot of room for individuality when I coach clients. For some people, doing the diet while on meds is the best foot forward. I applaud any movement in the natural direction. Everybody's path is different, including what does and doesn't help them feel good. I think that biochemical individuality—understanding what works for you and your body—is an important part of the human experience.

For example, a lot of people with autoimmune issues swear by probiotics. Personally, I spent thousands of dollars on them with no visible results. Later, I learned that as long as there's inflammation present in the gut, you really can't repopulate it with probiotics. It's like a hot furnace down there—any good bacteria you send to your intestine are just going to be annihilated by inflammation. (Wish I would have known that before I spent all that money.)

By contrast, people who eat a variety of colorful veggies and a diet high in soluble fiber are going to be in a state of constant, gentle detox. There's less of a need for repopulating the gut with probiotics because they aren't killed off as quickly, and a healthy diet will feed and care for the ones you have.

This bio-individuality principle is an important thing to consider when you're a parent of a kid with Crohn's. You can have two kids with the same parents and one ends up with strange stomach issues, while the other doesn't. Go figure. Same parents, same food, totally different sensitivity makeup.

The good news is that children tend to respond quickly to these changes in diet, much more quickly than adults. What's more, by coaching them on this diet, you'll be setting them on a path they can follow the rest of their life—a path of being healthy and understanding how food affects their body.

Bear in mind, though, that the Desperation Diet isn't

an easy diet for adults to follow; good luck with the kid. It's definitely worth the battle when you can know for sure that it works, and that you're not pumping your vulnerable child with medications that have the potential for long-term side effects. But I won't sugarcoat it—it's a challenge for parents to help their kid follow this healing diet, because you can't reason with them on an adult level. (Not that adults are all that easy to reason with, either.) For most of us in the developed world, the food we eat isn't about reason, is it? It's about taste versus what the body needs.

> My own daughters watched me struggle with Crohn's, and I still have a hard time getting them to eat as much soluble fiber as I think they need. Kids want to eat what their friends eat. Teens in particular are like a little herd of amoebas, all looking to each other for acceptance. Even if it makes them double over in pain after they eat it, they'd rather eat the food that everyone else is eating, than something that could help them feel better.

There's nothing like Crohn's to help you understand that the food you eat isn't just about what it tastes like—it's about what it's doing for your entire body. Everything we eat either is supporting those fifty trillion cells, or it's not.

If you don't want to eat what's good for you all of the time, that's fine. But if you commit to redeveloping your lifestyle around healing food, you'll actually be able to retrain your taste buds. Instead of being assholes, they'll become your allies. Imagine that!

Discover How Great It Feels to Say "No"

Healing from Crohn's makes you look at your life so differently. For thirty-four years, I was "healthy." I looked good, I could run and play sports, I could travel, I could go out and drink with my friends. I could do all of these things that we humans view as normal and fun. I had no idea that all of those things were aiding in a quiet nightmare building in my cells. There was no reason for me to know that—I was in the "invincible" stage of my life.

Crohn's really changed that conversation around health for me. It's not about what's "normal" compared to other people around me. It's about what I actually need to do for my body to work and feel amazing. I had to consider what real deprivation looks like—is it denying yourself a taste bud-pleasing treat, or denying yourself real nutrition and lifelong health?

This was the question that started the conversation with myself about how my taste buds are assholes. They want Cheetos and chocolates and a milkshake—all the things that have nothing but bad to offer my body. When they made a fuss about something they wanted, I started actually talking back to them: "You guys are assholes and care only about yourselves."

It was healing for me to be dedicated to this diet and what it was doing for my body. The day I could sit in a chair without needing to rock back and forth as a palliative for the pain, that was amazing. The day that I was able to walk my dogs around the block, that was huge. Those were some of my personal milestones that let me know that I was headed in the right direction.

It was also healing for me to start saying "no" to getting together with people. I got so tired of having the Crohn's conversation every single time I went out with people, that I just gave up doing it. I said, "You know what? I'm only going to hang out with people who know I have a sickness where regular food makes me shit my pants, and that will not give me a hard time for doing what I need to do to take care of my body."

Don't Be a Lab Rat Anymore

Research tells us that our health story is only 20 percent determined by genes passed down to us from our families, and 80 percent food and lifestyle. That means our health is 80 percent determined by our own choice! To me, Crohn's comes down to what I've done or what my parents have done to my body, i.e., medications, vaccinations, food quality, and life choices. I know, hunt me down like a crazy witch for even mentioning vaccinations. But just because everyone does something, doesn't mean it doesn't have consequences and long-term effects.

Sadly, humans have become the largest test market for the pharmaceutical industry, to our own demise. Many things passed as healthy or okay for human consumption years later have been found to cause cancer. If your goal is not just to get better, but to live a long, healthy life, you must commit to being your own health advocate. It's a little more work, but it sure beats being a lab rat for Big Pharma.

There's this common idea people have that we're either blessed with "good genes" or saddled with bad ones. We think that things like heart disease, addiction, or allergies are just genetic roulette. I've heard people say things like, "My dad could always eat/drink/smoke whatever he wanted, and he lived to age 85," assuming that their own body is exactly the same, as if bodies in the same family just rolled off like Xerox copies from the same DNA strand.

It's true that our genes do make us more or less sensitive to various factors. But it's not just our genes alone—it's what we do with them. How we live, how we eat, how we move. For example, every one of us has cancer cells swimming around in us right this moment. The question isn't whether we "get" the disease. It's whether or not our bodies express that gene. Hereditary traits make us more or less susceptible to that gene being expressed, but your diet and lifestyle are what pulls the trigger.

Let's say I have the gene for autoimmune disorder, that it's part of my family's hereditary makeup. My lifestyle is what determines how that gene gets expressed. If I take good care of myself, protecting myself from consistently high levels of stress and feeding my body the kind of nutritious fuel it recognizes and can easily use, it may never express that gene. After all, an autoimmune disorder can't really express itself if there's nothing to trigger it, right?

Which brings me to my special PSA for those not currently suffering from stupid autoimmune disorders:

A Note to the "Healthy" People Reading This Book

If you're reading this for a friend or loved one who has Crohn's, colitis, or suffers from stomach stuff, I'd implore you not to take yourself out of the equation as you read this. You might be "healthy," but consider making changes to your diet today just to safeguard yourself. Drop white stuff from your diet, and add in soluble fiber during your day. Realize that even that small stuff is going to help increase your chances of future health. I think that makes it worth doing.

If you start this while you're healthy, it's possible that you actually might feel worse for a little while, because your body is pulling out some toxic stuff. Push through it—it won't take long—knowing that it's aiding your body and making it more able to eliminate the foreign toxicity that lurks inside of you.

The younger we can start doing good for ourselves, the better chance we have of fighting off what we consider in today's world the inevitable disease. In every family, there are certain conditions or diseases that everybody just takes for granted—cancer, heart disease, diabetes, on and on. It's time to ask yourself, "How could I be the generation that stops that genetic progression in my family?"

Bottom line, good health is not a sacrifice. It's a gift. Don't waste it.

4

Making Your
Shit Work

. . . .

After lots of trial and error, what actually got my shit to work (literally as well as figuratively) was a super simple diet. Who knew that one simple, all-natural food would be all it took to cure my Crohn's? Not me.

But it took me some time to figure this out.

Any healing diet you can name, I tried it. The first and most obvious thing I tried was eliminating all highly suspect foods. Everything I liked—fried foods, gluten, nuts, candy, alcohol, dairy, red meat, soy—banished from my plate.

But that didn't fix my issues, and honestly, I didn't expect it to. I knew instinctively that my sickness went deeper than a common food allergy.

The next thing I thought of was going back to the hippie farmer-forager lifestyle of my childhood in Big Sur. Crawfish pulled from the stream, locally grown and wild vegetables, mushrooms and fiddlehead ferns foraged from the woods...all the amazing gifts from the dirt that fed my family when I was a child. I even considered going back home and eating some local dirt in hopes of getting some of my childhood microbiome back inside me. I didn't, though.

However, that ultra-clean, all-local approach didn't fix me, either. So I rolled up my sleeves and got to work, testing every popular "healing diet" I could find. I boiled down chicken and beef bones to make broth, and drank it by the gallon. I swallowed every probiotic I could get my hands on, both in pill form and in my food: kimchi, sauerkraut, this amazing fermented yogurt that I special-ordered from a tiny company in Texas. (Beyond that, though, all other forms of dairy, along with wheat and especially sugar, were banished from my presence.)

I thought for sure that if no single one of these approaches worked, a combination of them surely had to. And I was ready to live the most ascetic life I could imagine, existing on a diet of sprouted quinoa and water kefir if needed, just to feel like I was living again.

But nothing helped. I just got sicker. Stupid Crohn's. So picky.

Clearing Toxicity

Looking back, it's easy to understand why none of these diets worked: they asked too much of my intestines too quickly. Don't get me wrong; they are all super healthy ways to live, and I recommend them for anybody who wants to help their body function at a higher level. But they all have this one thing in common: they require lots of bile. And when your bile is toxic and your intestines filled with a foe called inflammation, even the cleanest, healthiest fat or protein means pain and suffering. I needed to clear out my body's toxicity before I could replenish it with all those amazing nutrients.

It's like being bitten by a venomous snake and expecting to heal while the venom is still in your finger. You have to stop the poison coursing through your veins before your body can regain its normal function.

Each time one of these healing diets failed me, I felt just a bit more broken. I felt like each failure was a point in favor of the doctors who insisted that my body was attacking itself—that I was crazy, and they were right. My body was just broken, and there was nothing I could do.

Nevertheless, I persevered. I don't know if it's my deep love for life, or my fierce (some would say stubborn) spirit, but I had (and still have) this sense of there being ultimate wisdom in the natural world. Something in me knew that there was a simple, uncomplicated, natural answer out there—one that didn't involve years of medication or several feet of my intestines being removed. It was that core belief that kept me going.

I'll keep repeating the fact that I love doctors. I really, honestly do. I believe that there are doctors out there who truly have a talent for helping and healing. Others are just emergency agents, and that's okay. Both are needed in today's world.

However, the sad truth is that a lot of Western medicine is oriented toward viewing every situation as an emergency in need of a quick fix, versus a situation that can be addressed in ways that contribute to longevity of health. While medical technology is racing forward at the speed of light, the knowledge and protocols haven't been updated in a long time. We're using fancy new tools to do the same outdated procedures.

My father raised me with the idea that there are healers in the world—people who love and intuitively understand the human body, who go the extra mile to understand what the body really needs in order to heal optimally. These would be the kind of people who work on vintage foreign cars, who take the time to really understand not just the machinery, but also its history, where it was built, where it's been, and what special treatment it might need.

Every now and then, you run into a doctor who is one of these healers. Someone with prestigious medical training who has that true reverence for the individual human body, who doesn't treat the cause of disease as an unsolvable mystery ("Your body just decided to attack itself") and solutions as one-size-fits-all ("Take this pill, and if it doesn't work, take two of them, plus this other one for the side effects").

The human body is indeed a mystery in some ways, but it's not devoid of common sense. If you put natural things into it, you can have a good sense of what's going to come out. If you put chemicals in, you have no idea what you're going to get as a result or when it's going to show up.

All of the tinkering that humans have done with our food, our water, and our natural environment puts foreign stuff in our bodies, expecting our bodies to use this stuff in the same way that they use organic matter. The body is like, "How am I supposed to use this? I don't even know what it is."

Maybe humans didn't need such a high quantity of soluble and dietary fiber until this precise point in our evolution. Now that we're dealing with standardized vaccinations, chlorine, fluoride and other added chemicals in our water, pollutants in our air, pesticides and hormones in our food, parabens in the soap we wash in...well, that's a lot of toxic buildup, even for people who strive to live a pretty healthy lifestyle.

There's a saying you may have heard before, that comes from Hippocrates, the father of modern medicine: "Let food be thy medicine." That's where I kept going in my head. I knew that the key to my healing wasn't a pill made in a lab. Food, pure and simple, would heal me. I just had to find the combination that worked.

The Diet That Finally Worked

When my friend dropped off Karen's book on my doorstep, I was at the end of my rope. For about twenty-four hours, I stubbornly tried not to make eye contact with the book slumped against my wall. What could this woman possibly have to say that I hadn't already heard? But eventually, just out of cynical curiosity, I cracked it open.

It turned out this woman had a lot worth listening to. Her book contained an idea I'd never heard of: a healing diet that pulled out the "venom" by removing the toxic waste that was burning the intestines of Crohn's sufferers. Not only was this diet highly restrictive, but it was totally counterintuitive. It was based on one of the foods most people, even healthy people, prefer to avoid.

The magic ingredient?

Beans.

BEANS?!

Yeah, no. Not happening.

That was my first thought. Even healthy people avoid beans, because they cause gas, bloat your stomach, and make you fart like a mofo. Nobody with a stomach problem wants to fill up on beans. I was the victim of chronic pain, fatigue, and a shitting issue that had no end in sight. No way, no how was I going to add this ingredient into my already precarious situation.

I read through the book thinking, *This is a total crock*. But the more I read Karen's story, the more I found myself believing in her. She had dealt with autoimmune disorders firsthand in the only way worse than having one yourself: with her children. After receiving no help or positive direction from the medical community, she took it upon herself to figure out a cure. She realized that she might be the only one who would do what it took to save her family.

I related deeply to Karen's "mama bear" instinct to do anything it took to save her babies' lives. No mother would settle for "pretty good" when it came to finding a solution to a disease that could damage her children's quality of life. If she said this diet healed her kids, I believed her.

On top of that, there were stories of other Crohn's sufferers that this diet had healed. People who came to Karen with a smorgasbord of medications were getting off those drugs. People whose bodies had been traumatized by surgery were actually reversing the damage they had endured. People just like me were not only getting their lives back, but living them better and wiser than ever before.

Those stories stopped me in my tracks. I remember thinking, *If food can do that, food is truly powerful. I never gave it that much credit.* At that point in my disease, I felt crazy enough to give Karen's bean-based cure a try. This diet would be my last stop before giving in to the doctors' "cut it out and cover it up" advice.

When I called Karen for my first consultation, she walked

me through a layman's understanding of the science behind the diet she'd created. She explained that fats stimulate the liver and gallbladder to release bile. For an inflamed intestine, though, bile is like putting lemon juice on a wound. If you have Crohn's, or similar conditions like colitis and irritable bowel, eating fat is actually the worst thing to do. Your intestinal tract is like one giant open sore, and every single time you go for that fatty deliciousness that you think is going to be really good for you, you're throwing gas on the flame.

I was like, *Gee, that makes total sense.*

In addition, most dietary fiber is like a scrub brush. In healthy intestines, it's a necessity, but when you send it into inflamed intestines, it's like taking a Brillo pad to your sores. All of these wonderful fruits and vegetables and whole grains I was eating in hopes of healing myself? They were actually hurting me. (Goddammit, Crohn's!) Even protein is difficult on your intestines because it takes a long time and a lot of bile to break down.

Over the first several months of trying the Desperation Diet, I'd call Karen whenever I felt scared or anxious. I felt both often. It helped so much to talk with her. She had lived through the fear I was experiencing. In talking to her, I heard the voice of someone who had suffered through the hardest things a wife and mother can experience, and had found a way to survive and thrive.

To this day, I talk with Karen on a regular basis. When I started my practice as a nutrition coach, I told her I wanted to help spread her information. It was pure luck that my friend dropped that book on my doorstep. I don't want people to get as desperate as I was before they learn this information—I want it to be easy for people to find.

I call Karen's diet the Desperation Diet, but it shouldn't be that. If we make a few small changes in favor of health, there's no need to get that desperate.

Ready to get started? Okay—let's dive in.

Warming Up with the White Diet

For people as sick as I was, you can't start the Desperation Diet right away. When you're working toward healing your intestines, the first thing you need to do is lower your body's production of bile so that you're not constantly rinsing your inflamed gut with acidic fluid. I learned from Karen that the intestines grow a new layer of internal lining every three days, which means that every three days, you have a chance to reduce the inflammation in your gut. Removing all of the irritating foods from your diet and eating the simplest, easiest-to-digest food allows your intestines to begin their healing process.

That food isn't beans. As wonderful as they are, beans take a little more effort to digest than your body has to give when it's super inflamed. The easiest food for your body to digest, the food requiring the least amount of bile for breakdown, is white flour (or a gluten-free equivalent). No fat, no fiber, no protein—just simple carbohydrates that are a cinch for the body to absorb for energy.

I know most Crohn's-friendly diets advocate against gluten and dictate copious amounts of nutrient-dense proteins and fat. I'm all for these nutrients in a healthy person who can absorb them efficiently. But when your intestines are in a state of inflammation, you've got to give them the easiest possible material to work with. It takes a lot of bile to break down protein and fat, and in order to reduce the inflammation in your gut, you've got to stop recirculating and producing bile for a little bit. You need to put out the fire before you start rebuilding the house.

Eating only white foods is just a way to give your body a break from the constant onslaught of fat-based bile. Fat isn't easy to digest, and the more complex, fibrous foods you eat, the harder it is on your entire digestive tract.

Karen calls this beginning phase the "White Diet," and it can last anywhere from a few days to a week, depending on how much damage is in your intestines. If you've caught the Crohn's disease in the early stage, you'll probably only need one round of the White Diet. After dealing with Crohn's for two years, I needed about two weeks of nothing but the White Diet for my intestines to rest, recover, and warm up for the healing power of the Desperation Diet.

During the first six months, I'd have to go back to the White Diet periodically, when my menstrual cycle hit like a monthly hurricane. For whatever reason, when I was on my period, the inflammation in my gut would flare up like an angry beast. During that week, I would go back to eating white foods and lean protein and beans, until the flare subsided. I love knowing I can always go back to square one; it's my safety net.

> When you are as sick as I was, this White Diet is as counterintuitive as it gets. When you're ninety pounds, your only desire is to eat fat, and lots of it, just to get some meat on your bones. BAD IDEA. Trust me when I say you'll only cheat once on this diet to realize it's not worth it.

For me, following the White Diet felt super weird because

I was eating everything my mom taught me *isn't* good for me. I remember feeling, "Okay, this is void of any and all nutrients...how is this helping me?" But the fact that the white food was void of nutrients was exactly what was helping me. My body didn't need to throw bile into the game in order to break down the food I was giving it. Remember, in a healthy body, bile is a great thing. But for a compromised system like mine, bile only meant pain and suffering. I had to give my intestines time to rest before they could get into the hard work of recovering.

> Many autoimmune disease sufferers have probably been advised by their doctors to avoid gluten. Doctors told me the same thing, not because I had a gluten allergy, but because it's a common food allergen. But when I started Karen's diet, gluten was the only thing I ate for the first several weeks. And it helped.
>
> My doctors didn't have much reaction when I told them I'd added gluten back into my diet. I think by that time, they were like, "Okay, hippie. Do whatever you want."

The longer you stay on the White Diet, the longer the opportunity you give your body to heal. But no need to stay on it longer than it's useful, as your body needs all the goodness of proteins, fats, and fiber. After giving your body a break, you can begin to introduce soluble fiber, which requires a little more effort from your body, but has the benefit of absorbing all the toxic bile from your system and getting it out of there.

Most of the horrible man-made toxic foulness hangs out in our bile. The liver is pretty bogged down with taking care of our own metabolic waste, and it doesn't have a lot of time to figure out the twisted shit we humans create. Thus, without an appropriate amount of soluble fiber in our diet, it just keeps recycling in the bile and fucking up our entire system. But soluble fiber, a.k.a. beans, grabs that toxic bile and poops it out. Yay, beans!

Simply put, soluble fiber on an empty stomach binds with your bile. Bile is fat, and soluble fiber *loves* fat. Soluble fiber is the Crohn's sufferer's best friend. It grabs the bile in your bowels, absorbs that toxic-laden liquid like a dry sponge, and moves it through your digestive tract and out of your system. Thanks, beans, you rock.

Now, here's the fun part: when the soluble fiber shuttles the toxic bile out of your body and into the toilet, this signals your body to release new bile to rotate through the body. And your body naturally circulates bile *every twenty minutes*. That means every twenty minutes, you've got a new opportunity to grab a little more of that toxic mess out of your gallbladder. All you've got to do is swallow another tablespoon or so of beans.

And that's exactly what I did. While doing the White Diet, I ate a tablespoon of beans every twenty minutes and waited for the fiber to work its magic. I didn't think of it as food, so much as medicine. Only instead of swallowing pills made in a lab, I was chewing "food" pills made by Mother Earth.

Another key during the healing phase is to keep your body hydrated, rested, and warm. Along with doing the White Diet, you want to sip a lot of warm water and sleep whenever you can. Sleep and warmth equal healing. Think about how you care for a baby—you're doing the same elemental things for your intestines, until they have healed to where they can function like "adult intestines" again.

Within about three months, I noticed a marked difference. My bathroom sprints decreased, and I started to feel less nauseous. I began to have a little more energy. I would go twenty minutes without pain, then a few hours, then a full day. Without the toxic bile constantly recycling through my body, my intestines could start to heal. That's the power of m*therf*cking food, people!

How Does This Even Work?

It's time for me to explain to you why beans are the bomb! And no, not just a fart bomb like you've probably always thought of them. They are a life-altering-in-all-the-best-ways cleansing bomb.

Beans are packed with protein, complex carbohydrates, and beneficial vitamins and minerals—copper, folate, iron, magnesium, manganese, phosphorous, potassium, and zinc. All good things for a malnourished little Crohn's homie.

Beans are my hero. They should be yours, too. Simply put, I fucking LOVE beans. Can you blame me? Beans did something that doctors couldn't do for me. They healed my gut. They sucked the venom. They gave me my normal life back.

I think I can hear you protesting, "But beans make me bloated and farty!" Listen, the only reason beans would be hard to digest is if they aren't soaked and cooked properly. And the farting and bloating are usually just the result of those beans pulling the toxic crud from your body. The more beans you eat, the more enzymes your stomach will make to digest them, and the less you will fart. See? Your body is a lot smarter than you give it credit for.

I am proud to say that I farted like a master until my body was clean. I am even prouder to say that these days, I eat as many beans as I want, and farting is not one of my current specialties.

Here's the thing: for this bean-based healing diet to work, you're going to have to really love beans. Because beans are gonna take center stage while your body is in its healing phase.

Yeah, I know. Say what?!

No sugar, no oil, no butter...nuttin'. Stop whining. This is your life and the health of your body that we are talking about.

To start off, you'll do the White Diet for three days. If you are in really bad shape, like I was, you can do the White Diet for a longer time frame, while gradually adding in beans (but keep up the white stuff, too). It's void of anything good for you. But for now, it serves the purpose of giving your intestines a vacation so they can regrow their lining.

Here are some of the delicious items you'll be enjoying during the white phase, depending on your gluten situation:

- White bread
- Short grain "minute" rice
- White rice cakes
- Rice Krispies
- Rice Chex

- White loaf bread
- French bread
- Bagel
- English muffin
- Flour tortillas
- Pita
- Noodles
- Pretzels
- Saltines
- Cream of Wheat or Cream of Rice cereal

Maybe you're thinking, "That's not so bad. I love white bread and pasta." Not so fast. The White Diet only works if you're eating these white foods with nothing delicious on them. No butter on your toast or potatoes, no sauce on your noodles...no flavoring at all, except maybe a little sea salt. The idea is that you're giving your intestines time to heal by feeding them with the simplest form of energy your body can process. No fiber, no fat, nothing that could cause the inflammation to continue.

I know it sucks. But the good news is that the White Diet is your opportunity to give some tough love to your asshole taste buds. You're breaking their flavor dictatorship over your food decisions.

When it gets hard, just remember that being a slave to

your taste buds is what made you sick. You can also be sure that once you start adding flavor back into your life, you're going to appreciate it in a whole new way. You might even be surprised to find that your taste buds start helping you make good nutrition choices. (More about that in Chapter 6.)

If you can't eat gluten, find the gluten-free substitutions of white bread.

But whatever you do, do NOT introduce brown rice into the White Diet phase. Here's why:

At this stage in the healing process, as far as your intestines are concerned, you are a baby, eating the most easily assimilated food. The complex fiber in brown rice will only irritate your intestines right now—think of taking a scrub brush to an open blister and you'll get the idea. There will be time enough for beautiful brown rice dishes when your intestines are healed.

You're also going to drink at least six to eight twelve-ounce cups of room temperature or *warm* water per day. Warm water calms the gut. Do it. You'll thank me.

You may not have any bowel movements while you're doing the White Diet. It's okay. Sure beats the usual shit storm. You also might find yourself a little grumpy. Let's be real—super grumpy. You're going to be hungry, and you're going to be weaning yourself off toxic foods. Warn your friends and family to give you some space during the next week or two.

Finally, don't be freaked out if you lose another pound or two while doing the White Diet. I know that even slight weight loss can be terrifying for Crohn's sufferers who are already emaciated from malnourishment. Rest assured that, for most people, the loss of a few pounds isn't going to send them to the hospital. You'll gain it all back, and then some, once you get into the next phase of the diet.

Beginning the Beans

After three days on the White Diet, you can slowly add a little bit of lean protein into your meals, such as chicken breast, white-meat turkey, fish, or eggs. I was a big fan of white rice with a scrambled egg and some sea salt. Do *not* introduce dairy, however—not even the fat-free kind. Dairy products have a protein in them (casein) that is very difficult for the human body to digest. Healthy human bodies can even have a problem with it, so don't push your Crohn's situation right now.

You can steam, poach, or cook your protein in a dry pan; the key here is no fat in any form. Remember, the reason why we don't eat fat in the healing phase is because fat stimulates bile, and bile stimulates bowel movements. Less fat = less pain, cramping, and bowel movements. More fat = more diarrhea, pain, and suffering.

Next, you'll start to add in two tablespoons, six times per day, of well-cooked beans. If you are stronger than me, you can work up to eating a half-cup of beans, six times per day. (Any kind you like—personally, I'm partial to black beans.) You can eat your beans with meals or in between. And if you have a flare-up, you can reach for another tablespoon or two of beans, chase it with some water, and wait for the soluble fiber to work its magic.

After about a week on the Desperation Diet, you can add in a tablespoon of nut butter and use some olive oil to cook with. If that goes well, you can experiment with adding well-cooked veggies into your meals. (Yay, variety!) The best candidates at this stage are green beans, carrots, summer squash, peas. To keep easy on your digestive system, you're going for the baby food consistency here. Open up, here comes the train...choo choo choo!

If at any point your stomach starts to misbehave in any fashion with one of the steps, take a step back. You might find yourself just eating white rice, some oil-free scrambled eggs, and beans for a while. This is fine. I lived on that combo, on and off, for a good three months. Let your body tell you when it's ready to move forward to the next step.

The Proper Way to Cook Beans

When I was really sick, you can be sure that I wasn't preparing interesting bean recipes in my crock-pot. (Not that you can do anything very interesting with no fat, protein, or flavoring.) Instead, for me it was just open a can of beans, rinse them in water, mash and eat. Being the ultra-natural human that I am, at first I was like, "No way am I eating canned beans!" But even opening the can was a challenge—so canned beans it was, and I was even thankful for them.

If that's where you're at, no shame. Just make sure you're buying organic, fat-free canned beans. It's also a good idea to rinse them before you heat and eat.

As I started feeling better, though, I wanted to learn how to prepare beans myself. Not only is it cheaper to buy dry beans in bulk, but there was something comforting about preparing the food that was about to heal me.

If you've never cooked beans yourself, here's a little primer:

Start by taking two cups of beans and soaking them overnight. This helps release the phytic acid, which makes beans difficult to digest. If you wanna take it a step further, go ahead and sprout those mofos. Next morning, rinse the beans, put them in a big pot, and cover with water. Cook on medium-low heat; don't burn them. Don't add salt. Pull out a few with a spoon every so often to test them. There's no such thing as overcooked or too-soft beans... the more you cook, the more soluble fiber is liberated.

My Experience on the Desperation Diet

Karen's book recommends doing the White Diet for a three-day cycle before adding in lean protein and beans. But because my intestines were in such bad shape, I needed to do the White Diet for a lot longer than that. Every three days, I noticed that my Crohn's symptoms got less intense. The first thing I noticed was that I wasn't running to the bathroom every ten minutes. The cramping that I felt had become less frequent and intense. The pain from my intestines that constantly radiated up into my back and my neck also lightened up. Even though I still wasn't totally convinced that this diet would work, I was ready to keep moving forward.

After about four three-day cycles of the White Diet, I began adding lean protein and, soon after, beans into my life. I started eating them in "mash" form, basically like fat-free "refried" beans. I wanted them to be as easy as possible for my body to break down, so that I wouldn't even have to do the extra work of chewing very much.

I worked up to eating about a fourth of a cup of legumes six times a day with my meals, or in between. I would get up in the morning, eat a quarter cup of beans, then wait a while and eat some rice, dry scrambled eggs, and another quarter cup of beans. I would eat another quarter cup of beans sometime in the middle of the morning, either all at once or as a tablespoon every twenty minutes (timed with the twenty-minute recycling of the bile). I'd eat more beans at lunch, more in the middle of the day, more at dinnertime. If pain woke me up in the middle of the night, I'd get up and eat another tablespoon or two of beans.

After a few months, I was strong enough to stand up, follow a recipe, and put some time and care into my bean routine. Cooking beans became something between an art form and a religious ritual for me. I'd eat my bean-based meals and think, "Oh my God, I love you so much." I'd pour my soaked beans into the crockpot, cover them with water, and I may or may not have whispered "good night" to them a few times.

At the six-month point, a miraculous thing happened: I went to the bathroom just two times a day, like a...gasp!... normal human.

For anybody with Crohn's, you know that feeling like a normal human in the bathroom is your highest goal in life. And having a perfect poo is like nirvana. Even today, every time I go to the bathroom, I'm like, "Hallelujah!" I never thought I would have a normal bowel movement ever again.

If you're reading this on behalf of someone else in your life with an autoimmune disorder, you might be grossed out by all the shit talk in it. But let me tell you, there's no one you can talk shit with like other sufferers from intestinal disorder. (Think how happy you feel after you begin to recover from a bout of food poisoning. Having Crohn's is like living with food poisoning every day of your life.)

When I'm coaching someone with Crohn's or irritable bowel, we will go on in truly gory detail about poop. It's nice to talk poop with a fellow sufferer. When someone experiences a perfect bowel movement, we celebrate together.

A NOTE TO THOSE WITH TRANSIENT IB OR MINOR STOMACH ISSUES

You guys don't know how close you are to healing! I get that it's uncomfortable and debilitating, but you're not at the truly fucked-up point that Crohn's and colitis sufferers are at. You're truly sitting on the edge of being able to heal. Don't give up—follow the diet, make the small changes, and you'll be amazed at how quickly your symptoms can clear up.

For several months after that day, I held steady on a diet of rice, ultra-lean protein, vegetables cooked down like baby food, and beans. And my symptoms continued to recede. The last thing to heal for me was flaring around my ovulation. No matter how well I was eating, I would have to go back and do the White Diet around my ovulation time. Then I got through it (but at a quicker pace) and would add my beans, protein, and cooked vegetables back in. It wasn't until about a year into the remission of my symptoms that I stopped flaring around my period.

The Speed Bumps in My Journey

Healing through food was a long process, and there were definitely times where I felt impatient. At first, I was just so grateful to feel less pain, then little pain, then no pain for long periods of time. But as I started getting my energy back, it was sometimes hard to keep giving my body the time it needed to heal. My family would go out to eat, and I'd have to order my food like a real asshole. "Is this cooked in oil? Can the chef cook it without any fat in it? Please make sure there's no butter on it." The server would say okay, and then I'd take a bite and instantly know, "Oh, my God, they put oil in it."

Those little things in food that nobody else would notice are powerful triggers for a person with Crohn's or colitis. A spice, an herb, a little too much fiber, a tiny amount of fat—your body really is that sensitive that any of those things will put it on the defense.

I'd go home and feel not only so sick, but pissed off because I was really looking forward to having a restaurant meal like a normal homosapien. But I had to realize that I can't expect a restaurant to be as strict as I can be in my own kitchen. Solution? I just didn't go out to eat anymore. If I had to go out for a work function, I would just get a plain bowl of white rice and tell my colleagues, "Yeah, sorry guys. I'm trying to heal and this is all I can eat."

Part of the reason I call Karen's diet the "Desperation Diet" is because you really do have to be in a state of desperation to try it. It's not complicated or exotic in any way. Instead, it's boring, bland, and requires a complete disconnection from your asshole taste buds. It requires you to treat food as nothing more than medicine. BORING!

You can bet there were days when I fantasized about the flavors I missed. It would have been easy for me to make all kinds of exceptions and excuses for myself on the Desperation Diet, especially when I had to travel for work. Obviously, it's not very practical to travel the world with a suitcase packed with cans of beans. I could have said, "Well, screw it—being healthy just isn't convenient for my lifestyle, so what's the point of trying at all?"

Instead, I decided to find a solution that worked for my health *and* my lifestyle, and what I found was psyllium husk. This humble little supplement was something I'd always had in my pantry, but I always thought of it as something you take when you're constipated. I totally did not realize that psyllium husk was soluble fiber in its most basic form. Just a couple teaspoons provides enough soluble fiber to help move out one rotation of your bile. (We'll talk more about this in the next chapter.)

I started putting husk into little bags and carrying it with me everywhere. I would take it on the plane, ask the flight attendant for a spoon and a cup of water, mix it up, and shoot it down right before the plane took off. When I landed, I would do it again.

That one simple solution allowed me to be mobile again in my early days of newfound health, which was amazing. I could move freely around the country, a foreign city, or anywhere at all, without scanning the horizon for the nearest bathroom. The most amazing thing for a Crohn's sufferer is not having to care where a bathroom is.

Following the Desperation Diet faithfully means that your desperate days are numbered. In fact, the Desperation Diet is really just a portal into the lifestyle of delicious freedom that comes with natural, food-based healing.

I know how hard it is to be patient with your recovery. You've been feeling better, then you experience these little setbacks and think, "Fuck! Am I going to be this sensitive forever?" It's really hard to accept that a restaurant isn't probably going to be as careful as you need to be with your body. It's hard to choose between going out with friends, knowing that you'll have to order something boring and bland while they're all enjoying a meal, and just staying home because you don't want to deal with it.

But I promise, it gets better. So, so much better. Just hang in there, stay consistent and don't give up. You're worth the fight.

Life After Desperation

It's a magical day when you wake up and realize you don't just feel not like death; you feel *good*. You feel like you. You feel normal.

Then again, this is a new normal. The old normal got you sick—it's normal if you feel a little bit scared of food, at this point.

Rest easy—the new normal you can eat everything your body is designed to eat. Here's how you can get started:

- Keep eating beans. Lots of them. But don't combine them with fat. Beans bind with fat, and you don't really want that unless you are eating chili and don't want to gain weight, as those handy dandy beans will bind with a good amount of saturated fat of whatever meat was cooked into the chili. For example, don't combine a meal of beans with the healthy fats your body needs like salmon, avocado, nuts, or tons of olive oil. Beans bind with fat and shuttle it out of your body, which means you won't get the benefit of your body absorbing those delightful fats. I usually eat my beans with some lean protein, veggies, and awesome spices.
- Eat fresh veggies and berries. Your plate should be mostly veggies, a palm-size portion of lean meat, and,

if you desire, a whole grain of your choice. (If you are uncertain what a "whole grain" is, Google that shit.)

> Variety is the spice of life. If you think of eating veggies and picture a plate of raw carrots and celery, you're doing it wrong. Eat a big old variety of veggies. Eat them raw, cooked, sautéed, and in salads. Get into it and enjoy. I didn't eat a lot of raw food for the following year after I went into remission. My body still had trouble digesting raw. Salads had to wait awhile. The hardest part of healing is the constant desire to rush forward.

- Olive oil is the only fat I use, as anything that is hard at room temperature is a saturated fat. There's nothing wrong with saturated fat as such, but I prefer to eat my saturated fat in the form of grass-fed animal protein.
- If you need sweetness in your life (and who doesn't?), eat some berries, drizzle some honey or maple syrup on a bowl of yogurt, or if you are seriously craving indulgence, spring for a little dark chocolate. But whatever you do, do it in moderation. Sweet in big quantities is crappy for your longevity, not to mention your overall health and well-being. It feeds all the wrong bugs in your body.
- Eat lots of nuts/seeds. That shit is good for you. I eat about a cup and a half of nuts a day—it's my go-to snack. My favorite thing to do is hit my local co-op grocery store and buy a variety of nuts (one of them

salted), mix them together in a big bowl, and store them in big glass jars on my countertop.

> What do you do when cravings hit? Two things:
>
> If you're just hungry between meals, start by downing a BIG glass of water. Most the time our "craving" or hunger is just dehydration. Give it a few minutes, and if you're still hungry, go for a handful of lightly sea-salted nuts.
>
> If you're craving sugar, it means your body actually needs some nutrition...stat! Again, nuts are a lifesaver here. Nuts deliver a wallop of nutrients plus a warm, yummy sensation of satiety. You'll get all the nutrition your body needs, and you'll actually feel satisfied.

- Ditch the iodized "table salt" and eat sea salt instead. Sea salt is yummy and full of nutritional goodness. You might as well get some extra minerals while you're flavoring your food.
- Drink spring water, or else get a filter on your sink. Chlorine is toxic. Fluoride is, too. (Yes, even in small amounts.) Don't poison the entire organism of your body in hopes of avoiding a cavity. Your liver doesn't like filtering out all the little bits of poison you shove into it because a doctor told you the amount is so small it doesn't matter. IT DOES FUCKING MATTER.
- Move your body. I don't care what you do—just do

something. But don't do it so much and so hard it's fucking you up. That's just as stupid as not moving at all. Longevity is the name of the game, so before you head to a three-hour CrossFit session, consider how long you'll be able do this activity regularly before your body gives out on you.

Is This Diet Forever?

When I tell people about the Desperation Diet, they nearly always ask:

"Do you have to eat this way forever?"

It's a funny question to me—do I "have" to eat in a way that keeps my body healthy and whole? At the same time, I get where they're coming from. Nobody, not even me, would love the idea of eating only lean protein, beans, and white bread for the rest of their life. (Although if I had to, I would. No joke.)

The answer, then, is yes and no. In some ways, I'm still on the Desperation Diet to this day—now that desperation has gone bye-bye, I call it the Longevity Diet. There are still some rules I follow, but they're a lot less strict than, say, the protocol I'd have to follow if I'd gone the medication or surgery route. "Managing" Crohn's means organizing your entire life around coddling your still-inflamed intestines. Nope, I'll pass.

Instead, now that my intestines are fully healed, all I have to do is make sure they stay that way. To do that, I live by a few simple rules:

- I don't do "white" anymore. If there's rice in the house, it's brown rice or wild rice.
- I eat tons of vegetables—I believe that vegetables should be the biggest portion on your plate.
- I eat lean protein on a regular basis, in an amount about the size of my palm, and I make sure it comes from animals that are grass-fed and locally raised.
- I eat organic and as close to me as possible. Bye-bye, bananas shipped from Ecuador and coconut products from South Asia. Hello, strawberries, blueberries and lettuce grown ten miles from my house.
- I steer clear of sugar, which is an inflammatory substance no matter what disease you do or don't have. I don't even eat fruit in large quantities, simply because I know what works for my body, and sugar in any form is not one of those things. I love chocolate and peanut butter enough to do a face plant in them...and from time to time, I do. No lie. But I do it mindfully, not in huge amounts and not every day.

I should add that these rules haven't taken over the "asshole" role that my taste buds used to play. I follow them 80/20-style, which I'll explain more about in Chapter 5.

This is the diet I follow during regular, everyday life. But part of being a Longevity Diet means that it makes room for unusual or special occasions. Let's be honest—eating all kinds of food is a central part of our lives as humans. The Longevity Diet lets me go out with my friends and have a drink or even two. If I'm on a vacation in an exotic destination, I can sample the local cuisine. If a friend comes over and brings a beautiful cake she baked herself, the last thing I want to do is respond with, "Oh, thanks... but is it sugar-free?" I even went out for a burger and fries yesterday, and I didn't have any stomach issues afterward. But I'm not going to do it every day, because I know it's not great for my longevity of health.

We all know that a burger and fries isn't "good for us"... but how many of us know exactly why it's not good? Let's take a closer look.

To start with, even the best grass-fed burger usually isn't palm-sized. And it's definitely not served on whole-grain bread, with a huge amount of fresh vegetables. Instead, it comes on a fluffy white bun that kickstarts the blood sugar, and it's served with a side of delicious, insulin-spiking potatoes fried in crappy, artery-clogging oils.

Even the most organic, health-conscious burger joint isn't going to venture far off the beaten path. Because when a red-blooded American consumer like you or me goes out for a burger and fries, we want a god-damn burger and fries. And we *should* get one! ...Just not every day or even every week. Balance, my friends, balance.

A lot of people think making changes to live a healthier life means deprivation or becoming a crazy Californian (like me). They don't want to have to change their routine. They don't want to have to give up their favorite foods (just eat them less often). They really don't want to be different from their friends, or have to constantly explain why they don't eat shit and get wasted anymore.

Cry me a river. You know what deprived is? Being so fucking sick you can't enjoy your life. *That's* deprived.

I don't know about you, but I'd much rather have to explain my healthy eating choices to people than explain, say, that I couldn't come in to work today because the pain was so harsh standing up straight wasn't an option. Or why I have to run to the bathroom every ten minutes. Or that I can't sit in a chair without rocking back and forth because the pain in my intestines is so excruciating. Or... well, you get the idea.

Health is not about deprivation. It's about loving yourself so much that living a full, joyous, satisfying life is the standard. Living for health and well-being requires that you contemplate health on a cellular level that comes from—surprise!—feeding your body healthy proteins and fats instead of simple carbs and sugar. It means looking past your "fast metabolism" or slender build and making sure you're building a body you can live in, comfortably and happily, until you're a ripe old age.

My motto is that if you give your body exactly what it needs to build healthy, radiant cells that elongate your healthy life 80 to 90 percent of the time, then you can spend 10 to 20 percent of the time doing whatever makes you happy in the moment. Because I recognize that a long life that isn't happy is not worth it, either.

I like to scoop a little nut butter with a square of dark

chocolate. I like to celebrate a successful work project with a juicy grass-fed cheeseburger. I like getting a little twisted from time to time in the form of tequila. On the rocks. While looking at the sea. For me, this is all part of living life to the fullest, which was the whole point of trying to heal my Crohn's disease.

Eating for health doesn't mean I have to be a food asshole. A food asshole judges what other people eat. A food asshole is terrified of soiling their perfect, pure insides with tainted "normal" food. To me, that is no way to live.

At the same time, I'm never going back to the "Screw it, I'm healthier than average" approach to nutrition. I'm not going to ignore the fact that I know my body is better off when I eat whole, nutritious, organic foods. I've learned the hard way that the human body is amazingly resilient, but it's not invincible.

The truth is that our world is filled with toxicity. It's not just in the food we eat—it's in the air, the water, the things we touch with our fingers, the clothes we wear on our backs, even in the energy waves that move invisibly throughout our spaces. And over time, this toxicity builds up in our bodies, unless we take steps to get it out.

The more I continue to work with people who are not

well, the more I see health as a gift that you give yourself. Really healthy people aren't people who upend everything about their lifestyle overnight. They're the people who change their thoughts around how they treat themselves. Instead of taking their bodies for granted, they make up their minds to do something really good for themselves. They choose to stay in touch with how they feel, instead of ignoring their body's distress calls. They take action in small, easy ways that add up over time.

This diet doesn't just help with Crohn's disease. It helps with life.

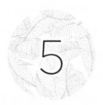

5

Other Shit That Works

· · · · · · ·

Karen's bean diet is what turned my life around, just at the moment I really thought my life might be over. But finding something that finally helped didn't mean my road to healing was always smooth. Even when you're on a protocol that works, even when you can tell that your overall well-being has turned a corner, there are bad days, frustrating surprises, and times when you start to wonder if all this effort is really worth it.

This is particularly true when it comes to the delightful array of mix-and-match side effects that come with auto-immune diseases. I'm talking mouth sores, skin issues, UTIs, yeast infections, rashes, and fistulas in all the most unglamorous places. Nothing sexy about autoimmune disease, people.

The reason for this comes back to where Crohn's shows up—in the small intestine. The small intestine is where you get all the nutrients that feed your entire body and keep it healthy. Having Crohn's means that, over time, your body is being slowly deprived of all the nutrients that normally should be maintaining your skin, your hair, your nails, your immune system, etc.

When you're seeking a Western doctor's help with Crohn's, they'll offer you all kinds of extra medications for these side issues. But if, like me, you're squeamish about pumping lots of shady pills into your body to "manage" your Crohn's, you're probably not interested in doing the same thing for all those Crohn's side effects, either.

That's why, in this chapter, we're talking about other remedies that work. Remedies that get you past the bumps in the road toward healing. Remedies that aren't going to stress your body out by introducing unpleasant side effects, but instead will soothe and sweeten your journey toward wellness.

Cannabis

Feeling nauseous all the time? No appetite for anything, including beans? I feel your pain—I was so fucking nauseous that drinking water made me want to hurl.

Fortunately, there are natural ways to deal with nausea and lack of appetite. You know exactly what I'm talking about.

For about six months, I took a hit off my bong before every meal. Hey, you can't heal if you can't eat the food that is supposed to heal you. And in my book, weed is a hundred times better than any prescription might-give-me-cancer-on-top-of-everything-else drugs. Bottom line, I'm totally well now, and weed helped the fuck outta me.

And in case you're wondering, I didn't trade out Crohn's for chronic as a way of life. I'm pretty much weed-free now; I don't feel the need for it. Now that I have radiant health, I'm high on life.

Baking Soda

Baking soda is a classic hippie remedy for all kinds of ailments, and not just because it's cheap. What makes baking soda so amazing is that it is highly alkaline, meaning that it neutralizes acid. Acid in large quantities stings, corrodes, and deteriorates.

This is why baking soda dissolved in water is a classic remedy for indigestion—it helps neutralize acid reflux. It's also why baking soda makes a great toothpaste, even all by itself. As kids, we used to mix plain baking soda with peppermint essential oil in a little bowl and dip our toothbrushes in it—it left our mouths feeling scoured and squeaky clean.

I often experienced indigestion while suffering from Crohn's. But I experienced instant relief by taking just a half teaspoon of baking soda in water. It's not tasty, but being addicted to "tasty" stuff is what got you here, right?

Moreover, baking soda is way better for you than the conventional remedies such as antacids or Nexium, which actually block your stomach acid and therefore block your body's ability to get all the goodness from your food. As a woman, the idea of not absorbing enough calcium was a huge red flag when it came to longevity. (Osteoporosis, anyone?)

> Crohn's sufferers often experience acid reflux. Believe it or not, it's usually not from too much acid. Acid reflux typically happens when the body doesn't have enough stomach acid to properly break down our food. Mind blown, right? Yeah, me too. So it's always a good idea to take a deeper look into your acid/alkaline balance before popping mystery pills. In the meantime, you could also try eating smaller meals, masticating like hell before you swallow, and possibly taking a digestive enzyme.

But where baking soda's healing powers really shine is in the bathtub.

I constantly battled UTIs while I was healing from Crohn's. The last thing I wanted to do was take antibiotics and kill the precious few beneficial bacteria left in my inflamed gut. So I looked for a natural remedy to keep my down-there system on the up-and-up. Lo and behold, I found one that really works!

For the baking soda sitz bath, you'll take about one and one-half cups of baking soda for four to five inches of bathwater in a standard sized tub) of baking soda and sprinkle it into the warm water as it's running. Stop the water when there's just enough to cover the area you're trying to heal. (This is a medicine bath, not a fill-it-all-the-way-up-and-relax bath.) The bicarbonate in the baking soda sends a negative charge into the water that will bind to the positive ions created by your body's acidic pH. (The baking soda ionizes in solution, allowing the bicarbonate molecule and sodium atom to travel into the orifices, i.e., the vaginal or urethra or bung openings). The bicarbonate and sodium ions are effective in killing viruses, bacteria, and fungi. That charge lasts for twenty minutes—about the time it takes to enjoy a magazine article, a podcast, or some soothing whale sounds. Sip lots and lots of room-temperature water while you're in there. At times like these, you wanna pee a lot.

After twenty minutes, the full effect of the baking soda sitz bath is complete. You can get out of the bath and go about your day...or drain the water and do it all over again. When I had a bad UTI, I would just stay in the bath, add more hot water and keep pouring on more baking soda, usually right where x marked the spot. Baking soda is completely safe and nontoxic, so I could literally do it all day, until I didn't feel pain anymore. Sweet relief.

It's really amazing how effective this cheap, natural remedy is. I've gotten rid of UTIs. I've gotten rid of yeast infections. I've gotten rid of sores. Oh, and I've gotten rid of a lot of the stress that builds up throughout a day of dealing with Crohn's. It makes you wonder how much better off we'd all be if we took 20 minutes for self-care like this on a regular basis. A candle, some Epsom salts and a lil' baking soda? I'm in.

In addition to infections and sores, I've heard from patients who have used the baking soda bath to relieve hemorrhoids, fistulas, rashes, you name it. I love hearing from people who start out doubting it and then call me to say, "Oh, shit, that baking soda bath was amazing... and it works."

The key with this remedy is catching your infection early. As soon as you feel that itchy, stingy sensation (or just suspect that something isn't right), clear your schedule for the next hour and jump in that bath. Fortunately, there are absolutely no negative side effects to this remedy. So even if it's a false alarm, the worst that can happen is you spent an hour sitting in the warm bath. Not a bad way to waste your time!

Garlic

Garlic is another home remedy that we all kind of know about...even if we don't know exactly why it's a thing.

Well, I'll tell you: garlic is nature's antibiotic. It's a powerful antioxidant with antimicrobial, antiviral, decongestant, and expectorant properties. While science does not have a full explanation for garlic's disease-busting effects, it's been widely shown to help the body kick some ass during flu season and beyond.

Even people who know this, however, tend to avoid using garlic medicinally. Just like beans, they think more about how it's going to taste (and smell on their breath) than about the many benefits they stand to gain. A pill, by comparison, seems a lot less messy. (Until the nasty side effects start showing up later.)

But when you've chosen to "just say no" to taking antibiotics, garlic is going to be your new best friend. And honestly, it's really not as bad as you might think. In fact, it can be pretty delicious.

I'm writing this in the middle of flu season. Everybody in my house is down for the count...except me! Twice each day, I crush two fresh garlic cloves into whatever I'm eating and down it goes. This isn't the most pleasant way to eat garlic, and I definitely stink, but damn, son, does it work!

Crushing fresh garlic causes a chemical reaction that releases allicin. Allicin is a powerful antibacterial that's only present right after garlic is crushed and before it is heated. It's not easy on the stomach; when I was dealing with Crohn's, I'd go small and steady with the garlic consumption, and make sure to eat it with food. Before long, though, my tolerance increased, and I was eating a clove or two of garlic every three to four hours.

That's still my approach for flu season and other times when heavy artillery is called for. But on a regular basis, I can take a more delicious approach to my natural antibiotic regimen. I slice up a whole onion and a clove or two of garlic, throw it in a pan with some olive oil, and cook them together until they are nice and brown and smell divine. Then I just add a few spoonfuls of the onion/garlic mixture on top of whatever else I'm eating—eggs, toast, rice, veggies and, of course, beans.

When you cook garlic and onion together, it creates a sulfur-rich compound that helps clear heavy metals, viruses, fungi, and mucus. If every human did that on a daily basis—cooked up an onion with the garlic and put it on the food that they were eating throughout the day—we would all be a bit more healthy and the smell would become the norm.

> Unsure of when to stick with cooking your garlic versus when to go raw? Easy. Raw garlic comes out when you're in a state of emergency and need to kill some shit you've already got, or if you want to nip it in the bud before it takes you down.
>
> Worried that raw garlic will upset your stomach? Don't start with two cloves like me. I've built up to that level. Start small—half a clove, chopped up and mixed into enough food where you don't taste it as strongly and it won't burn your tummy.

Hot Water

We all love to drink hot things when we're sick. Hot water is by far the best thing for your body when it's in a compromised, nutrient-deficient state. Your body absorbs warm (or even room temperature) water more easily than cold water. It hydrates you quickly, while also calming and soothing an upset digestive system.

I encourage every Crohn's sufferer to sip hot water throughout the day. No need to put anything into it. But if you'd like to liven things up or you want a yummy tonic to treat what's ailing you, here are my go-to tea options:

Ginger

Ginger is amazing for settling nausea and other stomach complaints, thanks to a bioactive compound called gingerol. (How original.) Along with being anti-inflammatory and antioxidant, ginger warms your body by increasing circulation.

Lemon

The side effect of almost any disease in the body is an acidic internal environment. When your body is extra acidic, it may seem counterintuitive to add more acid with something like lemon juice. But in fact, what tastes acidic to us actually has an alkalizing effect on the body. (By contrast, meat has an acidic effect in the body, which you'd never guess because it doesn't taste acidic. Go figure.)

Tonic Tea

When I've got a cold coming on, I'll combine all the above into a powerhouse immunity booster. Fresh ginger sliced thinly into a cup, followed by a healthy squeeze of lemon and a whole thinly sliced garlic clove. This will immediately clear your sinuses, thin the mucus in your system, warm your digestive organs to do their job, and keep the sickness from settling in your chest or your gut.

Psyllium Husk

When I first started learning about the health importance of soluble fiber, my natural first move as a mom was to get my daughters to start eating more beans. As you might imagine, they were a firm no go on that. After all, they weren't sick...why did they have to do the food-as-medicine thing?

Rather than fight with them over it, I found another way: psyllium husk. I'd stir it up in a shot glass and hand it to them right when they woke up in the morning. "Drink this," I'd say. "It's preventative medicine that will help your body stay healthy. If you like your body the way it feels now, take it." They were too tired and groggy to argue, so they'd just drink it and move on with their morning. Score one for Mom.

Even to this day, I can get them to take the psyllium fiber

at least once a day. I can't tell you how good it makes me feel that I'm giving them a little bit of a head start in living a healthier life, not to mention teaching them that health isn't all about pleasuring those asshole taste buds.

If you're tired of preparing beans, have a travel schedule like mine, or have other life obstacles getting between you and your soluble fiber needs, psyllium husk can be your other best friend.

It's tasteless, goes down easy, and takes just ninety seconds to measure, stir, and gulp it down. What you don't want to do is let it sit—the fiber will create a gelatinous texture in the glass that is no fun to choke down.

The best way I've found to take it is to mix up about a tablespoon of husk with a little bit of water in a shot glass, then shoot it down and chase it with a glass of water to drink. Better yet, make that two glasses of water to chase it. If you don't drink enough water after taking psyllium, the husk can have a dehydrating effect.

> Reminder: the reason why you take soluble fiber an hour-plus away from meals is because soluble fiber binds with fat. While you do want it binding with bile, which is made of fat, you don't want that fiber to bind with healthy fats that are carrying nutrients into your body.

Natural Supplements

The beautiful thing about the Desperation Diet is that it allows you to heal through food. That said, if there's a natural, whole-food nutritional supplement that works well for you, there's no reason to stop taking it.

> The same cannot be said for prescription medications, which can introduce more toxicity into the body even as you're eliminating toxicity through soluble fiber, and slow down your progress in healing.

For instance, I took a combination of Chinese herb preparations such as Isatis Cooling, Flavonex and RF Plus to ease my symptoms while I was doing the Desperation Diet. I found these herbs in the homeopathic section of my natural foods store, but you can find them online, as well. Aloe vera capsules were a lifesaver that cooled down my hot-as-hell intestines while I was healing. I used both for a year, then gradually weaned off them.

If you're interested in taking a supplement, do your research, consult a specialist, or visit a good natural foods store and talk to the person at the supplements counter. Even when you've chosen a good one, use common sense, and start slow. Taking the wrong supplement for you, or even taking too much of the right one, can be inflammatory.

Heating Pads/hot water bottles

I was freezing all the time when I had Crohn's, thanks to my weight loss and poor circulation. Being cold not only felt miserable, but it also slowed down my healing process. If you're not making a lot of energy already (because you can't eat food), being cold is very taxing on your body. And the more energy your body puts into keeping itself alive, the colder you get.

By contrast, heat is very healing for the body. It increases circulation, encourages detoxification, and by helping your overworked body relax, it encourages healing.

All these are great reasons to invest in a heating pad, especially a moist one. Mine became my best friend. I would sleep with it at night. I would take it on planes. Kidneys, chest, belly, back—every part of the body loves heat.

Stress Reduction

We've all heard it a billion times, right? Long-term health demands that you reduce stress in your daily life. Stress will corrode everything you count on—your energy, your health, your mood, your motivation—to power you through your life.

Despite all we know about the negative effects of stress, most of us keep finding reasons to stay stressed out and even add stress to our life.

I was one of those people—always on the clock, working like a crazy person, telling myself I had no choice. Without realizing it, I'd created an internal environment ripe for developing an autoimmune disorder.

Part of my stress came from being always on the go—up early, working late, traveling the globe. But the stress went a lot deeper than that. As much as I love people, my nature is more introverted—I'm most comfortable around one or two people whom I know well. However, I was ambitious to progress in my career, and that compelled me to say "yes" to a lot of needlessly stressful situations. I can remember getting through presentations in front of large groups, then returning to my hotel room and collapsing from exhaustion...only to get up a few minutes later to attend meetings for the rest of the day, and then "reward" myself with empty calories and alcohol.

Looking back, I can't believe how fucking crazy I was. I never stopped to acknowledge that it's not good for anyone to have that much adrenaline pumping through their system on a regular basis. Then you add in a nutrient-deficient diet, just eating whatever my asshole taste buds desired. Maybe without all the stress, my body could have handled the food choices I made better. (Big maybe.)

I thought I was being a badass, refusing to let my fear or insecurity get the better of me. It took Crohn's disease to help me realize that if I didn't prioritize my physical well-being above all, I wasn't going to fulfill any ambitions or goals I had for my life.

If I'd responded to Crohn's the way my doctors wanted me to—heavy doses of immune suppressants and the possibility of multiple surgeries, the chemicals of being put under multiple times, subsisting on multiple medications—that would have put my body under even more toxic stress. It might have held some of my symptoms at bay, but it would have created an environment in which my autoimmune disorder was being suppressed instead of healed.

I have a much better awareness of my stress levels now. I don't choose to override the signals from my insides that I'm getting nervous or uncomfortable. I don't allow myself to stay in a constant state of fight or flight. I know that I'll never accomplish my life goals if I let them take precedence over my physical health.

It's no coincidence that a high-stress lifestyle goes hand in hand with a high-caffeine, sugar-laden diet. I wasn't starting every day with a doughnut, or dumping Sweet'N Low in my coffee. But when I felt tired, I would make a cup of tea and add a few teaspoons of brown sugar. When I felt tired or grumpy or just needed a little pick-me-up, a handful of M&Ms was my go-to. And let's not overlook the other big sugar factor that most of us never consider: alcohol. Like most people, my idea of "relaxing" after work centered on a couple or five cocktails, or a nice bottle...I mean *glass*...of red wine. All that shit adds up, people.

The life I was living was pretty common by advertising industry standards—live fast, party hard, make money, and fit into those overpriced jeans. I was constantly in a state of stressful highs and lows and, unbeknownst to me, it was killing me. But if you'd seen me then, you would have thought I was just having a blast.

I'm still in the advertising biz today, even as I'm coaching people and working toward my nutrition certification. It's crazy to look around me at all the cute, energetic young people who are doing the exact same thing to themselves that I used to do. Everybody is going a hundred miles an hour, working around the clock, thinking, "I'm dedicated, I'm kicking ass, I only need few hours of sleep and then I'm up and grinding again." Meanwhile, I feel as though I'm watching this entire generation turn into unhealthy time bombs, right before my eyes. They will have so many fucking issues because none of them actually listen to their bodies. Their only "health" concern is making sure they look good. (Because being slender means you're healthy, right?)

In many ways, that stressful way of life suited my personality. I like to keep moving, and I'm a junkie for adrenaline and somewhat hummingbird-like in how I physically and mentally jump from one thing to another. The downside is that my emotional center is super sensitive, so I go into fight or flight pretty easily. If somebody says, "I need to talk to you," and I have no idea what the context is, I immediately become twelve years old again—*Oh fuck! What did I do?* I'm a lot better at not letting shit get to me so easily these days, but it still doesn't take much for my stomach to churn.

A lot of people live similarly, whether it's their natural state, or just their life circumstances. Everything from having a hectic schedule to routinely putting yourself through hard workouts can put your body into a catabolic fight-or-flight mode. And the junky things we put into our bodies certainly don't help.

For instance, we all know by now that coffee isn't great for us, because it puts our nervous system on the fritz and stresses our adrenal glands. But most people consume coffee because they like the taste, that little jolt, and the routine around it. They're not contemplating the fact that they're putting their body into a potentially unhealthy state, which causes the digestive tract to shut down, in order to avoid a perceived emergency. Staying in that mode all day, every day, creates a lot of toxic stress on your body, which can result in (among other things) digestive problems.

Soluble fiber is an awesome source to get rid of the toxins that build up in the bile and help regulate the overall digestive system. But it's also important to fend off stress through activating the parasympathetic nervous system. It's a healing stage that revolves around getting oxygen into your bloodstream. Fight-or-flight cuts off this supply, but things like deep breathing, yoga, and gentle exercise activate the parasympathetic nervous system, which helps you reap the full, healing benefit of the oxygen you breathe.

It might sound like a hippie thing, but making time to

pause and breathe deeply and intentionally is immensely healing. You don't have to meditate or even close your eyes. Just sit for five to ten minutes and breathe deeply until you feel relaxed.

We're in constant motion, never in this relaxed healing state. Relaxation is key to healing.

Patience: The Magic Ingredient

If you're like me, growing up in a natural household or just one where you were pretty open to trying home remedies, this "remedy" won't be too hard to swallow. (No pun intended.)

But if you're like the majority of Americans, you're much more comfortable with running to your local pharmacy for a flu shot or throwing down whatever pills the doctor puts in your hand. You might be reading this chapter and thinking, "Does all this *really* work?"

I get that skepticism. I really do. The whole thing with Western medicine is that it promises to fix things immediately. Make the pain go away *now*. Stop the discomfort *now*. Blast the sickness out *now*.

But let's be honest—is there anything in life that doesn't

come with some sort of consequence? Do you really think you can take drastic action on your body without having an equal reaction? Yeah, me neither. Just because the side effect doesn't come right away doesn't mean at some point in your life you won't have to pay the piper. Even something as harmless as taking a painkiller has a side effect.

My teen kid has a go-to response when I caution her about the potential long-term consequences of her choices: "That's a Future Me problem." But is it a Future YOU benefit? When everything is good, few people ever stop to think about what this immediate gratification is doing to their bodies as a whole organism. We never stop to question whether carpet-bombing our guts with antibiotics might actually make us worse off in the long run (i.e., sicker more often and for longer periods of time) than simply taking some down time to be sick and giving our bodies a gentle, natural boost to heal the way they're built to. Every choice you make today is either helping or hurting Future You.

As a kid growing up with ultra-earthy parents, I got so used to hearing things like "the Earth provides everything we need" and "honor your body" that I got bored of it. I felt deprived and would seek out junk food any chance I got. I wanted to watch TV and eat junk food like my friends. That attitude stayed with me well into adulthood, until the day that I found myself in a deep hole of sickness that I couldn't get out of.

Despite my best efforts to thwart my natural upbringing, my childhood was ingrained in me. When it came time to buckle down, I knew it was okay for healing to take time. It's okay to find something else to alleviate this issue while you're working on the biggest issue: returning the body to a healthy, non-toxic state.

Let me tell you, there's nothing like a doctor declaring that the only solution to your suffering is to prescribe gnarly meds and cut out a piece of your intestines, to make you consider trying natural alternatives. In that moment, the "honor your body" mentality I'd been raised with kicked back in. For the first time, I understood why my parents tried to raise us that way. Staying healthy was easier than trying to get healthy again after illness.

The quick solutions offered by Western medicine work by acting in extreme ways on the body. But every action has an opposite and equal reaction—that's just physics. You can pump antibiotics into your body to kill the bad bacteria, but you're also going to kill all the good ones in the process, leaving you with little to no immune system, and we now know that 70-80 percent of our immune system lives in our gut. (To say nothing of the importance of gut bacteria on things like fertility, mood, skin and hair health, and so much more.) What happens if you get a cold? Or eat something that disagrees with you? Or, God forbid, the bad bacteria grow back?

If somebody says, "This medicine will cure your illness, but it has the potential to blow out your pancreas," how is that even medicine? If they say, "Oh, don't worry—only one in every 500 people has that happen," I'm still not into it. I don't even want the possibility of blowing out my pancreas. To me, taking that premeditated chance is saying that it's okay with me if I become one of those 500 people. And it's *not* okay with me.

When doctors told me, "I can put you on this pill for this issue and that pill for the other issue," I would Google everything about the medication they were proposing. And wouldn't you know it, every medication they said that they could give me to make one thing go away caused another issue to show up. What sense does it make to "silence" one disease by poisoning the entire organism and quite possibly creating other issues?

With Crohn's in particular, if the standard medical remedies—medications, surgeries, etc.—actually made the pain and suffering go away forever, maybe there would be a reason to take that chance. But Crohn's sufferers have been following their doctors' orders for years, *and many are still fucking suffering.* I know one guy who literally has no intestines left at this point, because that's how doctors "managed" his disease. They continued to remove and remove and remove, until there was nothing left. And guess what? He's not all better. His anus is a colostomy bag. But he is alive, and I suppose that's something.

By contrast, the people who did the Desperation Diet are living pretty normal lives. Sure, like anything, it might NOT work for everyone like it worked for me, but for the most part, they're not in and out of hospitals. They're not trying different pills every month. They're free of active disease, and their health is their responsibility. Their only "life sentence" is eating well to keep a healthy body. And when and if a flare happens? They go back to the White Diet and thoughtfully contemplate what made them flare, so as not to go down that road again.

I know I've said it a billion times already, but I'm going to say it again: I love doctors. But doctors are, by and large, trained to do anything they can to stop the problem as soon as possible. That mentality is amazing in the case of an emergency. But when it's a chronic, ongoing issue, taking drastic action means (to me, anyway) losing control and not taking responsibility for our own health. I don't think it's fair to put doctors in the position of saving us from something we have most likely co-created through our food and lifestyle choices. I hated being in pain, but I understood pain was a messenger. It was my body's way of saying, "Dude, you fucked up." I understood that my body was looking for ways to repair whatever I'd inadvertently done to it in my fully unconscious state.

Having a doctor tell me, "Your body is attacking itself," sounded absurd to me. What could make my body attack itself for no reason after thirty-four years of behaving rationally? I had to figure out how to help my body help me again.

Yep, You Really Are What You Eat

It's a cliché, but that doesn't change the reality behind it. Your body takes on the qualities of what you put into it.

Everywhere I go, I look at people and want to knock the horrible shit they're eating out of their hand and say, "Dude, wake up! That shit that you think is amazing because it tastes so good? At some point, the Grim Reaper is going to come and require your gallbladder as payment."

We have so much variety, it's almost as if we don't know what to do with ourselves. We're like, "If it's out there, it must not be that bad." Never mind that it's full of Yellow

#5 and Yellow #6. Never mind that it's packed with sugar, the common denominator amongst nearly every chronic inflammatory disease. There's this sense of, "I can, so I will." Or even worse, "I deserve this as a reward for working so hard/having a hard day/being pretty healthy most of the time."

I'm not saying that you have to shun the warm, gooey works of genius at your local doughnut shop. I'm not saying that you should never take a trip down memory lane with a favorite food from your childhood.

But here's what I *am* saying:

Stop being a mindless food consumer. Start contemplating that your body is the vehicle that carries you to all of your most amazing moments in life, moments that can be savored for much longer than any meal. Those moments are worth being healthy for.

Making Healthy Normal Again

The thing that I really don't want to do with this book is put another hippie health manual on the market. I'm not a hippie. I live a very normal life. I don't live in a teepee on a remote mountainside, refusing to join modern society. (Though I'll admit that I secretly want to live in a yurt.) I have a lovely little bungalow, a nice car, and my two kids go to a good school. I use a cell phone and binge-watch my favorite Netflix series.

I shouldn't be considered a health-nut or a hippie because I give my body what it needs to thrive. I should be considered a mindful human who is taking care of her most prized possession.

I want this book to set the precedent that a normal person can and should call out the bullshit idea that we can eat whatever we want because it tastes good, or because we work hard and deserve a break from reality.

A happy, normal life isn't about the house. It's not about the car. It's not about the job. And it's not about being entitled to eat whatever you want as a reward for how "good" you've been in other ways. If you don't feed yourself properly, then everything you consider normal will break down. It's a matter of when, not if.

What so many people refuse to be honest about is that we co-create our health situations for ourselves. I co-created my sickness by making toxic choices, eating stupid shit, and seeking quick relief for every pain or discomfort I experienced. I never stopped to think that every choice I made could add up to a cumulative effect and pull the trigger on some unsavory genes. I just didn't know...or, more truthfully, I chose not to stop and acknowledge the obvious.

Normal people work out so they can eat what they want and look healthy. But let's not just look healthy. Let's *be* healthy. Believe me when I tell you that it's so much easier to stay healthy than to get healthy once you've been sick. But if you've taken that journey to get back to health, you can never, ever go back again to the way you were before.

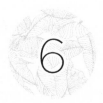

6

Nothing Tastes as Good as Healthy Feels (Sorry, Kate Moss)

· · · · · · ·

It's not about size, it's about content.

There are people who cut their disease out and go back to doing exactly what they did before. And then, oh my God, they have a flare-up. They go to the doctor and get another medication, thinking all the while, "If this pill doesn't work, we can always try another, or cut the diseased part out."

They do it this way because they don't know any better, or feel they don't have any better choices. They're thinking of their intestines as a single thing, not connected to a bigger whole.

Nothing could be more wrong. Your entire body is sick when your intestines are sick. Inflammation in the intestines is the result of sickness, not the cause. Cutting it out just takes away that specific area; it doesn't mean that the issue is gone. There is this disconnect between how far down the sickness spectrum you've found yourself, and what you were doing on the way there.

Organic Is for Wealthy Healthy People

Any person who drives a nice car knows that when they get to the gas tank, they're going to fill it with the highest-grade fuel they can buy. They're not going to get to the gas station and say, "Fuck it, I can't afford that. I'm just going to put this other shit in and hope for the best."

However, we follow that philosophy with our bodies all the time. We visit natural food stores or the local farmers' market and think, "Ugh, I can't afford to eat local, seasonal, and organic all the time. Why even try at all? I'll just hit the drive-thru."

What you need to know is that every time you choose the convenient over the nutritious, you're actually shortchanging your life by shortchanging your cellular structure. Every cell in your body is nourished by the food that you eat. We need healthy fats, proteins fiber, vitamins, and minerals to survive...and guess what? You're not getting those things out of thin air. You're getting them from your food. Your body deserves the healthiest, highest-grade food, just like a fancy car deserves the best fuel. Better fuel means better performance. Period.

I'm equally flabbergasted by the philosophy of eating shit food while taking vitamins. 90 percent of the time, your body doesn't even know what to do with vitamins. For the most part, those little capsules are just offering you single elements out of what naturally comes in a form your body understands—a whole fruit or veggie.

For example, vitamin C doesn't show up in nature all by itself. It comes packaged in a vegetable or fruit with fiber, vitamins, and minerals that also benefit your body, all of which help each other get assimilated by your body.

When we take vitamins in pill form, we're taking these elemental things and telling our body to recognize them as if they were the same thing we'd find in real food. They're not. Vitamins can be a great addition, but they should not replace good quality food. Food, my beautiful people, is our greatest medicine.

Just a heads up that most of the vitamins on the market are not whole food vitamins. In other words, not all vitamin C is made equal. You're just trusting that somebody made a good product for you—a product that is, by the way, unregulated. You have no idea what it is because they don't have to tell you. There's a lot of snake oil on the market. Do your research.

Taste Buds and Toxins

In Los Angeles, where I live, cleanses are a favorite topic of conversation. Even people who eat a standard American diet know that they have toxins in their body that they should probably get rid of. Every now and then, I'll hear a friend announce, "I'm doing a cleanse." Whether she lives on cold-pressed juice for a week, or does the lemon/cayenne/maple syrup cocktail, or some other version of the detox protocol, she's convinced that it will drain the bad shit out of her body and—fingers crossed—she will lose a few unwanted pounds.

A juice cleanse can be a great catalyst diet. If you've never eaten healthily a day in your life, a juice cleanse will give your body an amazing break from serving as a garbage can for your mouth. It can help reset your relationship with nutrition, and maybe even help get your asshole taste buds in line. However, I'm not a huge fan of juicing as a way of life. We really need to eat the entire fruit or veggie—all that fiber is needed to help slow the absorption of sugar in the bloodstream. Fiber is king. Without it, you're just filling up on mineral-rich sugar water.

After the juice cleanse is over, you might feel lighter from losing some water weight. You may have even shrunk your stomach a little. This is all great, as long as you don't let your newfound health stay skin-deep!

We are what we eat, which means you have the power to alter your health history. So if you go the juice cleanse route, use it as an opportunity to reset your taste buds. Break your cleanse with whole food shakes and add in some healthy fats, like nuts and seeds. Eat those fresh salads, farm-fresh eggs, and grass-fed meats. Eat local, eat seasonal, and honor your heritage in the healthiest way you can.

Your digestive system is your second brain. It runs every-thing in the body. If we feed it properly, it does its job effortlessly and we don't notice it, which is, of course, how we end up taking it for granted. We think, "I'm good. I'm strong. I'm healthy. I'm made from good stock."

I'm one of those "made from good stock" people. But I squandered it, and by the time I realized what I'd done, I was really weak. I was ninety pounds of nothing but skin and bone. My body had literally cannibalized itself because nutrients were so hard to come by. As soon as I would put something in my mouth, it would turn to water, and I'd be running to the bathroom with all this undigested food coming out of me. My joints swelled. My knees and fingers hurt—I'd wake up and my hand would be in a claw position. Nothing worked properly when my intestines weren't working properly. It was a steady decline. My body didn't have enough nutrients or fuel to run the organism, because it was too busy fighting a level of toxicity that no juice cleanse could alleviate.

Teaching Your Taste Buds to Be Health Buds

The minute you start thinking of what you eat as an opportunity to feed your body nutrient-rich materials, all of a sudden, your taste buds' influence comes to a screeching halt. You instantly stop craving the shitty food and start craving the foods that heal and help you.

Just kidding, it's not that easy. Haha, sorry. Each day you make a choice to stay healthy and make better choices, and some days are easier than others.

However, it is possible to change your taste buds from assholes into allies. You don't have to fight them forever. You can actually train them to be "health buds" that crave the taste of nutrients. Yes, really.

Thanks to the many months I spent using food only as medicine, my taste buds underwent a complete reset. I started tasting the subtle flavors in the vegetables I cooked, the creamy richness of farm-fresh eggs, the nutty sweetness in brown rice and beans.

Today, my taste buds have become my homies. They discern what's really in the food I'm eating. I can't even handle the taste of food that is chemically processed anymore. I'll put something in my mouth and instantly spit it out. Even with things like alcohol, and my beloved chocolate, my health buds will throw up a hand after just a bite or two—"We're good. More than that just isn't going to be beneficial."

It's a great day when you know that your taste buds are now working for you, rejecting things that they know aren't going to do you any good. Nothing feels better than knowing you can trust your taste buds to fight for the better interests of your body.

Of course, even on a good day, when you smell some old familiar junk food favorites, your taste buds might get confused and say, "Oooh, I want that. I deserve it. I *neeeed* it."

But instead of obeying whatever they tell you to do, you'll

have control over your choices. Now you know that as soon as you swallow whatever they want, your body is going to have to make sense of it and most likely pack it onto your ass, because it doesn't know what else to do with that nutrient-deficient cloud of shit. Ten minutes later, because you didn't give your body any actual fuel, it's going to be hungry again.

The human body is built to fight off occasional parasites or infections from wounds or bouts of food poisoning, but not to process man-made chemicals on a regular basis. Our bodies can only fight off illness if we're living in a normal state of health. If we're not, then the parasites and diseases get in, and our body is like, "I can't fucking fight this off. I don't have the resources to maintain a healthy balance of good microbes to battle the bad ones. And because you're taking a PPI all the time, you're actually suppressing my hydrochloric acid, so I can't kill off your parasites."

Some people might protest that we live longer now, and it's proof that all this toxin talk is hippie shit, and our diet can't be *that* bad. In fact, the real reason for our increased longevity is more likely to be the fact that we finally invented indoor toilets. (It makes sense that while people were throwing their poop out into the street, life was shorter.)

But then, only a couple centuries later, people were like,

"Hey, let's create Wonder Bread. It's cheap, convenient, and lasts in the kitchen for years." During those times, a lot of quick fixes were invented to help the working mom get food on the table in a hurry. People were trying to just survive in the short-term, so there wasn't a second thought given to the possible long-term effects of these chemical pseudo-foods that were basically void of all nutrients.

In reality, the human body needs what it has always needed. It needs healthy grass-fed or wild protein. It needs a variety of fresh vegetables and fruits. And, of course, it needs a way to get what you don't need out of your system.

That's where your "good bugs" come in. Say hello to my little friends!

Meet Your Microbiome

The human body is made up of more "bugs" than human DNA. Let that bend your mind for a bit. From mouth to tail, skin to feet, your insides are covered in bacteria. They all communicate with each other, the outside world, and the bugs in your food, and it's the communication of these bugs that actually helps maintain our homeostasis. Our human body communicating with the invisible world around us. When you're healthy, the good bacteria inside your body outnumber the bad bacteria, and the food you eat helps maintain this balance. The good bacteria within you are also outside of you, in healthy soil and water and air. How beautiful is that?

When you take an antibiotic, you're not simply curing an infection. You're killing off part of your internal biome, your first line of defense against germs and invaders. Even if you take probiotics afterward, do you really expect to replenish your entire body of bacteria from a few strains in a capsule? It's a beginning, but it's not the answer. The answer is to act preventatively and try to alleviate yourself naturally, if at all possible.

We need to slow down and look at the bigger picture of our choices. There's this common overreaction to our bodies. Got a headache? Take a pill. (Not drink some water or cut down on caffeine or change your diet.) Instead of rushing to get rid of the pain, take a look at the pain—what could be causing it? Our body doesn't enjoy randomly causing us pain for fun. There's always a reason. If we take the time, we can train ourselves to hear what our bodies need.

Obviously, in the moment, most of us can only think about making the pain go away. It's time to change our philosophies around "fix" to "inquire." Calm down, and find out what the body is telling you. Symptoms are your body telling you that something you're doing on a regular basis isn't working for it. In this situation, pain relief is actually a bad thing, because it's helping you ignore something that your body needs to tell you about your lifestyle. If you silence your body, it's going to shout at you louder and louder. Covering up that small pain now is almost a guarantee of greater pain later. Constant becomes chronic.

I don't know when we as a culture got to the point that suffering was never okay. It's a bummer to suffer, but that is a natural part of our life. We are so quick to stop discomfort without asking why our body is doing what it's doing. When I have a fever, I rarely take anything for it. I know that a fever is simply the body's way of eliminating the invader germ, virus, or bacteria. I stay hydrated, rest, and keep an eye on the thermometer to make sure I'm still within a safe range. (Nobody's trying to be crazy here.)

My rule of thumb is that antibiotics should only be used when totally necessary and only when they are truly the only answer. Stay home and get some rest—that's why we have sick days, people.

If you have a raging infection, you're peeing blood, or you can't breathe easily, deal with it. Don't be an idiot and just sit in a baking soda bath. Call 911 and get some emergency help.

But if you haven't gotten to that point yet, pay attention.

If your body is throwing you messages, listen to it. Deal with it before it becomes an issue for which you need an emergency intervention. Respecting our bodies means actually listening and responding thoughtfully to the messages they're sending.

Dedication, Not Medication

When someone comes up to me and goes, "Oh my God, I heard you cured your Crohn's naturally—how?" I settle in. I love supporting those in need of a little health guidance or support. I want to be an inspiration for those fighting for something good: their health and longevity.

I know how scary it is when you're sick. You just want to run away and try to find a quick fix, instead of going through it slowly and steadily. You don't have to climb the mountain alone. And as much as you might want to, you can't really go around the mountain. Cutting it out and covering it up is a Band-Aid that will eventually fall off. Healing takes time. You gotta go through the mountain. Do the work. Make the changes.

If you've been suffering from Crohn's for a long time, you may feel too tired and disillusioned to try another thing. I feel you. Maybe at this point, the idea of baking soda baths and drinking warm water and eating beans for every meal just feels like too much, and you'd rather just take a pill. Maybe you're exhausted with the search for what's going to work, and this feels like too many different things to keep track of.

Dedicating yourself to a healthy way of life is not easy, especially in a world where we've never had to dedicate ourselves to anything. People quit school, jobs, marriages, and families because they get bored or it's too hard. Healing, like all good things, takes time.

If you're in a state of emergency, you're going to do whatever it takes to get out. But when you get out, contemplate how you can support your body by giving it what it needs, so that your amazing vehicle can heal and can take you to all of the places you want to be in life.

For me, a big part of this change was changing my mentality around the idea of a "treat." I grew up defining it as something I put in my mouth: "If you eat all your dinner, you get a dessert." When you're treating yourself, it releases those happy endorphins associated with reward and happiness. But how is that really a reward or a recipe for happiness if it's hurting your body in the long run?

I needed to change the mentality of "I'm going to treat myself" to something more like, "I'm treating myself to extra longevity and richer life experience, because I have a healthy body and a healthy mind." (Don't worry, I just punched myself in the face for you.)

But it's true. I want to treat myself to being an older person who doesn't need fifteen medications to get up in the morning. I want to treat myself to living 100 lives within a lifetime, and to experience all kinds of things at every age.

Define Yourself Through the Lens of Longevity

As a child, I was never afraid or in denial about death. I knew that I wanted to die having lived an amazing life, having seen my grandchildren, having reached the goals that I dreamed about. It wasn't just about happiness in the moment. It was about the entire picture of human life—I wanted to have a rich existence, to deeply experiences all the ups and downs that make life amazing. At the end of that story, I wanted to die peacefully in my bed.

Now, having been sick, I realized my childhood goal was always about longevity. Not just how do I reach an old age, but how do I really *live* to that age?

I was thirty-four when I got sick. That point was my wake-up call; I was like, "If I actually want to be that older person who dies in her sleep after living this amazing full life, I'm not going to get there the way I'm going now." Not only I was burning myself out physically and emotionally, but I was literally burning up my intestines with inflammation.

The Desperation Diet put me back on track toward fulfilling that childhood fantasy of dying as a happy person who lived a full life. I could have done this diet and then, once I was feeling better, gone back to an overindulgent life, with everything I ate being about my whims and my passions and what tastes good now, while telling myself that anything less would be deprivation. But you know what? Giving my body what it needs so it can give me what I need, changing my thought process from deprivation to celebration of all the memories I have yet to make and all the things I have yet to learn, feels like a MUCH wiser exchange. Life is meant to be lived, and live I will, thanks to my amazing, resilient body. Longevity of health tastes better than any "treat" you can buy at the store.

Really Enjoying Life

I remember my daughter saying to me once, "Mom, why would they make it if it were bad for you?" I remember looking at her and thinking, "Oh my God, I wish humans cared for each other like that." I wish humans did make things that were only good for each other. I wish that, when you pick up a candy bar, it came with the warning label that said, "This could aid your body in creating more cancer cells."

I recently heard some crazy stats that within every human body, we already have cancer cells living there—it's just a matter of whether our T-cells are able to fight them off or not. The reason why there's more and more cancer showing up is because our lifestyle and food choices are weakening our body's immune system and its ability to protect us. Think about that: It's not that we could "get" cancer. We already have cancer. It's whether or not we cultivate it. Mind blown.

Why should "enjoying" life consist of indulging in things that are bad for us? Life isn't just about eating and drinking whatever we can get away with. It's about so much more.

Yes, it's fun to indulge occasionally in food or drink that you love. The key is consciously contemplating that choice: "If I am not going to give up my coffee, how am I balancing the rest of my life? How am I going to give my body the things that it needs so that, if I desire something beyond what my body needs, I can have it without stressing my body out?" When you've made a conscious choice to indulge, you're able to enjoy it so much more.

Personally, I pretty much gave up the majority of alcohol in my life...except for tequila, which is obviously the nectar of the gods. When I'm out with my husband or friends, I'll occasionally choose to sip a shot of tequila. I want to have fun and get loose and enjoy my night with people. But there is no reason for me to wake up the next day feeling like shit, just because I didn't listen to my body's signals to stop.

I know people might resist what I have to say. "Oh, this diet you're describing sounds too restrictive. I don't want to be a slave to a certain eating pattern." Fine, but do you want to be a slave to the limitations of your body, once your unhealthy eating habits catch up with you? At least with this diet, you get to make that choice. You don't just wake up one day and find that you can't sit upright in a chair without rocking back and forth. I've been there, and I'll tell you this: it's a way more restrictive way to live than not being able to eat anything my asshole taste buds tell me they want.

I find it surprising that so many people are more comfortable cutting pieces out of their body, or covering up their dysfunction with a pill, than they are with the idea of imposing their own restrictions on themselves. Especially when taking a pill or cutting it out doesn't actually ensure healing! I would rather do something that I personally control, instead of letting doctors go in and cut something out. Once that happens, you surrender control. You don't know what the scar tissue is doing in your body. You don't know whether if, for the rest of your life, that point where they sewed you back up is going to bleed forever.

Instead of silencing your body, why not try acknowledging that it's saying something to you? Why not stop and listen for a change to the truth inside you? Your body isn't out to hurt you. It certainly isn't attacking you. It's trying to heal you and help you live. Isn't that what you want? Why not give it a chance?

Conclusion

You're Great

. . . .

Let's say I said to you for the rest of your life you can't eat sugar anymore—if you do eat it, we're going to have to remove your pancreas. How many people do you think would say, "Just remove my pancreas?" The idea that "life without sugar (or coffee, or alcohol, or fried food) is not worth living" just doesn't compute with me.

Life without health is the one that's not worth living. I can give up sugar, I can give up coffee, I can even—sigh—give up alcohol, if I need to. But the one thing I will never again give up is my health.

I can say that with certainty because I'm on the other side of a horrendous disease that left me on the floor, crumbled into a million pieces, sobbing. I was in so much pain. I was so depressed. I was so unhappy. Worst of all, I could remember what it felt like to be well, to be normal, to love life.

Everybody who knows me would tell you, "Oh my God, nobody loves life more than Unique." I love life, I love people, I love the hard times as much as I love the good times. It's all beautiful.

But I went from being that person to a person who every night asks to just die, because I was in so much pain and it seemed like there were no options for me. Everything I tried failed, and the suffering was constant.

My healthy body today is a reminder that disease isn't worth mindless living. Health is the ultimate gift that we give ourselves. Health is what allows me to fall in love and to love another person and to inspire other people and to connect with other people and to hug other people. Health is the gift of all gifts, and one we can give to ourselves. Talk about self-love.

If you feel mostly fine and don't feel like there's anything you need to change, you have nothing to lose by trying the Longevity Diet. But if you feel like you're too far gone or too deteriorated, you really have nothing to lose. You either get healthier in some respect and make some strides toward the better side of the street, or you don't. Either way, you have nothing to lose. Trust me when I say there is no downside to making some longevity tweaks to your diet. It's valuing yourself to do what your body needs so that you can continue living this amazing life, whatever that looks like for you.

Information is free. Everything I've said here can be found on the internet or in another book or brochure in some nutritionist's office. We don't change because of information. We change because of transformation—a point coming in our life that inspires us to want to change. I'm hoping that the simplicity of this content is an occasion for such a transformation.

It's really the process of questioning our thought process around why we choose the things we eat. When you order food, why do you order it? What are you looking for? Why is it one of your favorite foods? Does it feed you on a soul level...or better yet, a cell level?

How much of what you eat do you consider is actually good for you? Not just flavor, but content. You are what you're made of. Every time you open your mouth and shove something in, that content is making up your cell structure. Scary, right?

Are you building a house that is strong and sturdy and

can stand the test of time? Are you building a house that's going to start crumbling and falling apart? What are you building? We are not invincible—what we put into our body matters.

It's time to really evaluate your thoughts around why you think you can or cannot change. Stop asking yourself whether you are strong enough or telling yourself that you aren't strong enough, and know that you are immeasurably strong. Besides, it wasn't my strength that got me to where I am—it was my determination and dedication.

Passion is something that can run out and fall on the wayside in life, but your determination and dedication is something that is constant. If you want to heal, then do it. You can do it. You definitely know that you can't just keep living the same life you've lived and expect different results.

It's really exploring the thought process around doing this diet and mentally preparing yourself. *Hey, this isn't going to be easy, and that's okay. Shit might even get worse before it gets better.* The things worth doing aren't necessarily the easy things. Healing isn't the path of least resistance. You have to face a lot of your own thoughts and beliefs to heal. Dig in; get real. You can do it.

Are You Ready?

If you're coming to this book ready to find something that works, but this big change feels like more than you can handle right now, it's okay. Changing overnight happens one bite at a time. It's a whole lifestyle switch, and that will take time. One of the biggest things you'll need is a good support team around you—a health coach, doctors who support your path, friends or family members who can help you explore your thoughts and really start weighing out what's more important between your taste buds and the health of your life.

The first thing to evaluate is your thought process around food. Most people would rather take a pill than feel "deprived" of all their favorite foods, or even just the ability to eat whatever they want, any time. This idea of deprivation needs to be addressed for real healing. Think about it—what do you want to heal for? Do you want to heal because you're tired of taking pills or getting an infusion? What is your reason for wanting to do this diet?

My reason for wanting to be on this diet was to assume responsibility and take control of my health. I also wanted to reconnect to my longevity as a human being. But there's a greater purpose in that than me just enjoying my time on this earth. I want to give back. I don't want to just take up space.

When you're sick, you can't give back. I believe the course of a human life is to give back, whether it's just to your own friends and family members, or to the next generation. It's to pass along hard-earned wisdom.

With this diet, I want to inspire people who are sick to heal, not cover it up and cut it out. I want to inspire healthy people to contemplate changes they can make today to continue being healthy and have an amazing, healthy, long life.

What I'd hope to give today, tomorrow, and forever is the message that taking care of yourself is worth more time and effort than you're giving it now. We're not just a vehicle for taste bud pleasure, but a vehicle for change, love, and community.

About the Author

· · · · · · ·

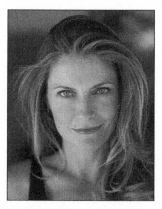 **UNIQUE HAMMOND** is a Crohn's survivor, nutrition student, author, health coach, wife, and mother who has helped countless individuals discover natural wellness and live healthier lifestyles. This Big Sur girl loves beach days and watching the sunset over a tumbler of tequila in her hometown of Los Angeles, California. To learn more about Unique and her refreshing, no-holds-barred approach to whole-body health, visit YoureGreat.com.